An Ordinary Future

An Ordinary Future

MARGARET MEAD, THE PROBLEM OF
DISABILITY, AND A CHILD BORN
DIFFERENT

Thomas W. Pearson

UNIVERSITY OF CALIFORNIA PRESS

University of California Press
Oakland, California

Library of Congress Cataloging-in-Publication Data

Names: Pearson, Thomas W., 1978– author.
Title: An ordinary future : Margaret Mead, the problem of disability, and
    a child born different / Thomas W. Pearson.
Description: Oakland, California : University of California Press, [2023] |
    Includes bibliographical references and index.
Identifiers: LCCN 2023001488 (print) | LCCN 2023001489 (ebook) |
    ISBN 9780520388284 (hardback) | ISBN 9780520388291 (paperback) |
    ISBN 9780520388307 (ebook)
Subjects: LCSH: Mead, Margaret, 1901–1978. | Children with
    disabilities—Legal status, laws, etc.—United States. | Children with
    Down syndrome—United States. | Parents of children with
    disabilities—United States.
Classification: LCC HV888.5 .P437 2023 (print) | LCC HV888.5 (ebook) |
    DDC 362.4083—dc23/eng/20230314
LC record available at https://lccn.loc.gov/2023001488
LC ebook record available at https://lccn.loc.gov/2023001489

Manufactured in the United States of America

32 31 30 29 28 27 26 25 24 23
10 9 8 7 6 5 4 3 2 1

For Michaela,
always,
and Aidric and Zora,
a remarkable future awaits

Contents

Preface

"I love you too, Dad."

She softly whispers it, like butterfly wings, orange ovals with black borders against blue sky and thin white clouds. Those are the last words I hear from Michaela every night, after the bedtime routine with her and her two siblings, after pajamas, after brushing teeth and reading stories.

In the summer of 2021, Michaela is six years old, our days packed with all the joys and trials and mundane moments that accompany parenting three children. Summers in northwest Wisconsin invite stunning beauty. The long, bitter winter, a seemingly endless season of snow-covered landscape, melts into an explosion of green, hillsides thick with trees and plants and insects, birds calling to each other, monarchs visiting wildflowers that burst with color. On days like this I love to take the kids on a bike ride. It's an adventure, really.

A journey.

"Time for an epic bike ride," I tell them.

My partner, Tiffani, a university event coordinator, often has a heavy workload in the summer, and leaves the house early. After a pancake breakfast, too much TV, and what seems like a never-ending ordeal of getting dressed for the day, we pack snacks and water bottles and head out to the garage. I take a few minutes to connect our trailer to my lime-green road bike, steel-frame with knobby tires and drop handlebars. I've been pulling my children with it since my son Aidric, now eight, was one year old. The back tire is pretty much bald and every year I tell myself it's time to replace it. These days, Aidric rides his own bike while Michaela and their sister Zora, now four years old, ride in the trailer, a red, canvas shell with torn plastic side windows and large black wheels. As I connect the trailer to my bike and load our stuff, the kids scurry about. It's hard for them to contain their energy. Aidric and Zora hop on scooters and shoot down the driveway. Michaela grabs a balance bike and bolts off after them.

"Stay in the driveway," I bellow. "No street!"

They turn into the street.

"Watch for cars," I call out with a resigned tone.

I keep an eye on them from the driveway as Aidric leads a quick loop of the cul-de-sac. Michaela goes up a neighbor's steep driveway and then turns around when she reaches their garage. She loves to cruise down, feet lifted into the air, and she comes flying back into the cul-de-sac to rejoin Aidric and Zora.

"Has someone checked the mail?" I ask, to lure them back.

They race to open the mailbox that stands at the end of our driveway. When they return, we put on our bike helmets and the girls get into the trailer. I buckle them while Aidric grabs his bike.

Some of our longer rides take us about four miles to Wakanda Park, located in Menomonie, where we live, on the north side of Lake Menomin, a former mill pond on the Red Cedar River. We take a bike path that wraps around a 3M manufacturing plant, farm fields, open prairie with long grass and blooming flowers, and eventually over an old railroad bridge converted into a bike path. We look for turtles and birds and deer and listen to the hum of traffic from the nearby interstate highway, concealed by trees. We approach a playground that sits atop a wooded bluff overlooking the lake, immense pine and oak trees shading the entire area.

"Wakanda, yea!" yells Michaela as we approach the park on our bikes. "I want that one!"

I'm not sure what she is pointing at. Probably the entirety of the play-ground, the whole experience, the thrill, the freedom, the closeness. The kids dismount and remove their helmets, tossing them aside as they run. They play on just about everything, but Michaela really loves the swings. She begs me to push her, and it must be a certain way. I stand in front of her, the two of us facing each other. I reach down and grab the sides of the swing she is sitting on. Then I step backward, pulling her with me, lifting her higher. She grasps the chains tightly, eyes gleaming. I lean back and count: one . . . two . . . three . . . rocking with each number, becoming more dramatic with each, then lifting her as high as I can before letting go.

Pure joy.

"Wheeee," she shrieks as she swings backward, away from me. As she comes back toward me, I reach out and gently tickle her sides. She laughs uncontrollably, her delight infectious. Nothing bad in the world exists in this moment. "Stop it, Daddy!" she says playfully. Zora and Aidric run over and want me to do the same. Michaela insists I push them too.

Eventually we hike around the wooded bluff. Near the top, a few hundred yards from the playground, a plaque embedded in a small boulder marks the location of an indigenous burial mound, "probably created by the Dakota or Sioux," it says, and thought to be over a thousand years old. Dozens of such mounds were excavated in the 1950s by an archaeologist and a team of community volunteers, a frantic salvage anthropology effort conducted over the course of a week. Construction of a hydroelectric dam would soon expand the lake and flood the mounds, and the earnest volunteers dug with the sound of bulldozers inching closer. The remaining mound is now part of a disk golf course that unfolds around Wakanda Park. On any given day, college kids trample the hallowed ground as they toss frisbee-like disks into metal chain baskets. At least once or twice a summer I walk out to the burial mound with my children to reflect on life, to talk about peoples who came before us, and to contemplate the hidden stories of the past. It is a brief encounter with the forgotten historical violence that shapes the present, a reminder of work still to be done.

"Show me happy," Michaela says suddenly.

She reads the consternation in my face. Perhaps more so than her siblings, Michaela is emotionally attuned to those around her. I guess I look glum.

I smile back at her. "I'm just thinking."

"Now give me hug," she responds.

And with that delightful embrace, she brings me back. Back to what is before me, and we resume our journey.

1 Becoming

Margaret Mead must have taken the call with excitement, expecting to offer congratulations. I imagine her delight quickly dissolved into dismay.

On the phone was Erik Erikson, at the time a little known forty-two-year-old child psychologist practicing in Berkeley. Born in Vienna, he had been trained in psychoanalysis by Anna Freud and came to the United States as Adolf Hitler began his brutal ascent to power. Erikson's work with children at the Pine Ridge Reservation in South Dakota, and his later collaboration with anthropologist Alfred Kroeber among the Yurok Tribe in Northern California influenced his theory of personality formation, which emphasized an individual's journey through developmental stages over the course of a lifetime. Each stage involves resolution of an existential crisis, as individuals reconcile their psychological needs with social expectations. His book *Childhood and Society*, published in 1950, would rocket him to international renown as an author and academic. At the time of the phone call, Mead and Erikson had known each other for years, connecting over their shared interest in the role of culture in shaping childhood and the socialization of children into adults. Erikson's wife, Joan, a Canadian dancer and artist he had met in Vienna and his lifelong collaborator, was expecting the couple's fourth child.

Hearing Erikson's somber tone, Mead would have pressed the phone against her ear, listening intently.

Joan had just given birth to a son they had named Neil. It was 1944. Franklin D. Roosevelt would soon be elected to a fourth term as president of the United States as World War II entered its final year. Like other social scientists of the time, both Mead and Erikson participated in research and writing for the war effort, with Mead contributing to national character studies and Erikson analyzing Hitler's rise to totalitarianism, a psychology of Nazism.[1] Joan's labor had been difficult, Erikson told Mead, and surgery followed. She was still heavily sedated. The doctors, he said, had just given him unexpected news.

Your son, they told Erikson, suffers from "Mongolian idiocy," a reference to what is now called Down syndrome. The baby should be put away.

In that era, it was routine for doctors to recommend that "mongoloids" be sent to special institutions. They told parents like the Eriksons that their babies would likely die before reaching two years old. That they would never learn to read.[2] Raising a mongoloid would sap the mother's emotional energy, her constant fatigue and detachment becoming a psychological burden for the other children, the normal ones.

Unsure of what to do, Erikson phoned his friend Margaret Mead.

After they encountered each other in 1934 at a month-long conference in Hanover, New Hampshire, just a year after he came to the United States, Erikson became close with Mead as well as with other anthropologists such as Ruth Benedict, both of whom influenced his thinking on identity and personality.[3] Mead was known for questioning norms and challenging authority. As a young woman in the late 1920s, she left her first husband and travelled to Samoa for research as she completed her PhD at Columbia University's Barnard College. A young American woman traveling by herself across the Pacific Ocean to study an exotic culture was a newsworthy endeavor, comparable with those of other trailblazing women who charmed the public imagination, such as Amelia Earhart. Her field research became the basis of her 1928 book *Coming of Age in Samoa*, a cultural analysis of adolescence that explored the sexual lives of teenage girls. Based on the relatively carefree experiences of Samoan teenagers, she argued that the sexual angst experienced by Americans was hardly universal or determined by human biology, but rather a product of cultural learning. The provocative book quickly became a bestseller, launching Mead's career as a famous intellectual. An adventurous image of Mead took shape in the public imagination: bushy hair cropped just below her ears, parted down the middle with bangs curving like crescent moons around prominent cheek bones, slack cotton dress with short sleeves and large pockets near the hip for her notebooks, its open collar revealing pale skin drenched with tropical sun. The image is one of a gentle, contemplative White woman sitting among dark-skinned native children.

By the time Neil was born, Mead was a giant in the blossoming field of anthropology who had cultivated an uncommon celebrity. *Coming of Age in Samoa* was followed just two years later with *Growing Up in New Guinea*, establishing her as a pioneering anthropologist and expert on the role of culture in the psychological development of children. It is through childrearing that something anthropologists had only recently started calling "culture"—the learned behaviors, norms, and beliefs that make a people unique—is transmitted from one generation to another. But childrearing practices also form a window into how shared cultural values and beliefs become imprinted into the personality of individuals. In 1942, she published *And Keep Your Powder Dry: An Anthropologist Looks at America*, solidifying her status as an anthropologist who studied unfamiliar peoples to reflect on and challenge her own culture's way of doing things.

Over the years, Mead had become a "strong, guiding female presence" in Erikson's life.[4] When Erikson called her, she was not only a friend, but also an expert who could offer a unique perspective on the crisis he was facing. As perhaps the best-known student of Franz Boas, the German-born scholar who had reshaped American anthropology in the early twentieth century, Mead embraced a broad understanding of what it means to be human and was intimately familiar with the varied ways in which families are formed across cultures. She and others in the Boasian circle, such as Ruth Benedict and Edward Sapir, also challenged the racial and biological explanations of human difference that dominated in the United States and inspired the atrocities of the Nazi regime in Europe. Mead is still remembered today for championing alternative ways of being human, for a fervent tolerance of diversity and respect for humanity in all its forms.[5]

She also tested the limits of Western cultural norms in her personal life. In an era when women were expected to fill conventional roles as wives, mothers, and homemakers, Mead was an independent professional who married and divorced three times and cultivated close, intimate relationships with other women, including Benedict. When Erikson called, she was the mother of a four-year-old daughter, a child with her third husband, Gregory Bateson. She famously drew on her cross-cultural experiences to challenge American childrearing norms, which in the 1940s emphasized rigid schedules and discouraged breastfeeding, and Benjamin Spock was her daughter's pediatrician.[6] *If anyone could advise Erikson, it would be Margaret Mead.*

Send it away. At once. Institutionalize the child, Mead told Erikson.

Don't let Joan get attached. If Joan were to hold her newborn, even one time, or even see it, the ordeal would be more difficult for her. Caring for a mongoloid would be damaging to the other children and the family's stability, Mead reasoned.[7]

Neil was gone when Joan regained consciousness. Erik informed her of what happened. Then he went home to his three other children. He wanted to protect his family, but instead he had planted the seed of a shared psychological trauma that would haunt them for decades. Neil's sister, Sue, was five years old at the time. "I anticipated the arrival of Neil with a special excitement," she recalls in her memoir. "Mom and I were to share something very special. I imagined that I would be needed and would earn Mom's love and approval by helping her with the baby's care. I would learn from her how to be a mother, and we would be close."

"Dad arrived to give me the news," she continues. "His face was anguished. The baby, he said, had died at birth."[8]

I am both an anthropologist and the father of a daughter with Down syndrome, so this story hits me close to home. I have wrestled with that same impulse to reject my own child, to deny her basic humanity. And I have turned to my training in anthropology, with mixed feelings about what I found, to help resolve the emotional turmoil.

For me, it began in February 2015. Barack Obama was still president and the world felt like a predictable place. The previous fall, a wave of unrest had swept through Ferguson, Missouri after the death of Michael Brown at the hands of the police, propelling the Black Lives Matter movement to national consciousness, but the upheaval remained localized, a story in the news. Donald Trump had yet to announce his candidacy for the following year's presidential election and was best known for his reality TV shows. I had been teaching full time at the University of Wisconsin-Stout for five years and owned my first home, an early twentieth-century Craftsman with a covered front porch extending the width of the house, where I lived with my partner, Tiffani, and our two-year-old son, Aidric. Having been at Aidric's birth, I was calm the second time around. I knew what to expect. Perhaps Erikson had felt the same naive confidence.

I accompanied Tiffani to the birthing center in the evening, returning home briefly to put Aidric to bed when a friend arrived to look after him. Tiffani labored most of the night. We walked the empty, dim halls of the small rural hospital, chatting about the past, about the future, pausing now and then when the pain gripped her. Early in the morning the labor progressed sufficiently and the doctor, a local family practitioner, was beckoned from his home. He rushed into the room, hair disheveled from sleep, to guide Michaela into the world. The nurse lifted her onto Tiffani's bare chest, and I saw a newborn embraced by her mother for the first time. Tiffani lightly stroked Michaela's forehead, her index finger tracing the creases on her brow, gazing at her with a mixture of adoration and exhaustion. I marveled at the raw beauty of it all.

Later, the nurse invited me to assist with measuring Michaela, a hospital ritual for new fathers that helps solidify their role. I picked up Michaela and nestled her close to my body, thinking she felt a bit limp or floppy. I even remarked that she seemed "light," but the nurse simply ignored my comment. This nurse had been cheerful and welcoming the day before, but now barely made eye contact as she briskly went about her work. I placed Michaela on a scale and straightened her legs while the nurse measured her length. I then pressed an ink pad against the bottoms of her feet. Her footprint was undeniably adorable, with a cute little gap between her first and second toes. The nurse stared at the print. After that I spent hours holding my daughter, peering into her scrunched face, stroking her tiny fingers and hands as she slept, gently rubbing my thumb into her palm. She had puffy cheeks and small ears, almond-shaped eyes, and her round head seemed to disappear into her shoulders. I was falling in love.

I had a faint suspicion in those early hours, nothing more than a muddled feeling, an inkling that something was not right. Michaela seemed different than Aidric had been as an infant, and the nurse's cold demeanor nagged at me. But the signs were subtle, and if others noticed, nobody said anything—not the delivering physician, none of the nurses, not even the pediatrician, who examined Michaela and told us she was perfectly healthy. My parents had driven six hours from Chicago and were the first extended family to meet Michaela. My dad commented on her "Asian eyes," picking up on the epicanthal fold that made her eyelids appear slightly slanted. I scoffed at him for being racially insensitive and explained that her features would smooth out after a few days. Infants are all scrunched up at first, I said. A friend who is a doctor and works at the hospital visited and held Michaela. A couple days later, we brought her home.

After our first night home, I found myself Googling "Down syndrome." I was sitting on the toilet with my iPad. I don't know exactly what prompted me to type the words, but I recall with striking clarity the moment I hit the search button. The internet expelled its findings, including many callous medical definitions that describe Down syndrome as an "abnormality" or "birth defect." I read about the "atypical" characteristics, the underlying chromosomal "disorder," and the inevitable developmental "delays." My breathing slowed even as my heartbeat quickened. I clicked on images and studied seemingly unusual traits—low muscle tone, upward-slanting eyes, small ears, flattened facial profile, a single deep crease across the center of the palm—many portrayed through the crude, somewhat inhuman sketches used to illustrate diseased conditions on medical websites. I read that the wide space between Michaela's first and second toes is considered a "sandal gap deformity," visible by ultrasound on "abnormal fetuses." But our ultrasound had shown nothing awry—or at least the technician had not noted anything.

I walked slowly upstairs, iPad in hand, contemplating with trepidation how to address this with Tiffani. The wooden stairs groaned with every reluctant step. I stopped midway on a landing to gaze out a window. Now and then I fall prey to preposterous doubts about my own health. In my mid-thirties, I experienced chest cramps when running, and quickly went to see my doctor, who ordered a battery of tests. He did so out of precaution. I have a thin, athletic build, exercise regularly, and had never had a serious health issue. He knew I was fine and confirmed that it was all in my head. In the two years since our son was born, I had redirected my irrational health worries toward his wellbeing, experiencing periodic episodes of halting anxiety that clouded my judgement. But I had to share this with Tiffani, I thought. I inched into the bedroom where she was nursing Michaela and noticed her computer open in her lap. She had tears in her eyes. I looked at her screen. She was already reading about Down syndrome.

That day we were scheduled to bring Michaela back to the birthing clinic for jaundice treatment, a common condition among newborns in my family. When we arrived, Tiffani immediately shared our suspicions with a nurse, who only then revealed that the possibility of Down syndrome had been discussed with the doctors after Michaela's birth. She told us they couldn't agree at the time whether lab testing, much less a diagnosis, was warranted. Since the physical signs weren't blatantly obvious, they had decided they would wait until the one-week check up to say anything, just to be sure. But now that we were asking about it, the nurse called the pediatrician, who immediately ordered a blood draw.

They would need to count her chromosomes.

.   .   .   .   .

Tiffani and I sat shoulder to shoulder in a consultation room, Michaela in my lap. The examination table was directly across from us, a wide strip of clean, white paper pulled down over the light blue cushions, a metal cabinet beneath. We undressed Michaela until only her diaper remained. I stood up and placed her on the table, resting my hand on her chest as the paper crinkled beneath her. Technicians tried to find a vein in which to insert a tiny needle, first in her arm, then her ankle and feet. It's tricky, with infants. Bright light illuminated the cold room from the ceiling.

Down syndrome results from a chromosomal condition that occurs during fertilization, when reproductive cells come together into a new cell to set the stage for human life. As the new cell divides, subsequent cells package pairs of chromosomes, one copy from each parent. Chromosomes are in the nucleus of cells, and each carries a single molecule of DNA, the instructions for how a living creature will develop. Most people have twenty-three pairs of chromosomes, for a total of forty-six. The diagnosis "Down syndrome" describes an extra copy of the twenty-first chromosome—three chromosomes rather than a pair—an arrangement known as trisomy 21. The trisomy occurs at the moment of fertilization. Scientists first discovered it only in 1959 and they now understand how it transpires (a process called nondisjunction), but not precisely why. Trisomy 21 accounts for 95 percent of all Down syndrome occurrences, and less common chromosomal arrangements such as translocation and mosaicism account for the rest. Roughly six thousand children are born each year in the United States with Down syndrome, about one out of every seven hundred babies.[9] While incidences tend to increase with maternal age, heredity is not a factor in trisomy 21, nor are environmental conditions. Its appearance is random, occurring around the world and throughout human history. Like many things in nature, there is no *why*, no specific reason the trisomy happens. It just does—a variation of chromosomes in the entanglement of biological reproduction and cellular formation. It is a natural part of the human condition, part of the diversity of humankind.

To make a diagnosis, they first needed Michaela's blood, dark liquid pulsating into small glass vials, which would be taken to a lab for analysis. The lab would produce an image of her chromosomes, called a karyotype, allowing them to be lined up and counted. Before the ability to visualize human chromosomes, for example when Neil Erikson was born, all sorts of wild theories were offered up about the cause of Down syndrome. Some nineteenth-century observers speculated the condition represented a reversion to a previous stage in human evolution, brought on by disease or even personal failing. By the early twentieth century, hereditary explanations were common, even as some scientists began to speculate that chromosomes had something to do with it.

As the vials were collected, the pediatrician talked about physical features, comparing Michaela to me and Tiffani. That extra twenty-first chromosome, repeated in trillions of cells throughout the body, shapes the array of characteristics commonly associated with Down syndrome. Older children or adults will often appear shorter in stature and have a round build, a wide neck, and a flat facial profile, but these qualities are usually more subtle in newborns. The appearance of an epicanthal fold, which my dad had picked up on, may give a distinctive eye shape. Low muscle tone is common, but this was not overly pronounced with Michaela, and doctors and therapists often remarked about her relative strength. In addition to distinctive physical characteristics, children with Down syndrome are at a higher risk for some health issues, such as congenital heart problems, but there was no sign of this either. The pediatrician also noted that she didn't have a "simian crease" on her palm, a single line running across the palm of the hand, as opposed to three creases.

I glanced at the palm of my own hand, pondering the curious reference to primates and the implicit transgression of symbolic boundaries that distinguish humans from other animals. The pediatrician's focus on the presence or absence of seemingly alien features left an uneasy feeling, creating distance, nudging Michaela toward a category that separated her from us, from normalcy.

"What do you think?" I finally asked.

"Hmmm. If I were a betting person," the pediatrician responded, "I don't know, but I would bet against a diagnosis."

It would be days before any lab results came back, perhaps an entire week. I sought refuge in denial. I'm not a gambler either, but I no longer had a choice—the dice had been thrown, tumbling across the table. I went to work but avoided my colleagues and tried to lose myself in teaching. I did not bring baby pictures to share, nor stories of Michaela's birth. I think the only person I told was my older brother, Jim. I texted him and asked him not to tell anyone until we knew for sure. At night, with Michaela and Tiffani up in our bedroom, I slept alone on the couch downstairs. I was separating myself, keeping Down syndrome at arm's length. I am not a religious person, but I prayed for Michaela to be "normal."

And I secretly hoped she would die.

.   .   .   .   .

At the time, like Erikson, I simply couldn't envision a future with Down syndrome. Dreadful thoughts flashed through my mind: Perhaps she won't survive these first days, sparing us all. This veiled "death wish," if it could even be called that, occupied my dreams in my rare moments of fretful sleep. They were abstract, ephemeral fantasies, really, my psyche conjuring scenarios that would somehow save us from what felt like an imminent nightmare, liberating us from the supposed challenges that lay ahead. The thoughts tormented me at unexpected moments, creeping into partial consciousness when I changed Michaela's diaper. I would stand over her, studying her features—her eyes, ears, the back of her neck, the shape of her head—yearning to discern the future like a fortune-teller reading the lines on a palm.

Tiffani is strong and typically stoic, but one evening she burst out crying.

"I don't think I want this," she said, sobbing. "This is not the life I want."

In the six years I had known her, I had never seen her cry like that. I tried to comfort her with tepid expressions of support.

"We can do this," I said. "Together." I didn't really believe what I was saying.

"I know we can do this," she countered. "That's not what I said."

Want and can are two different things. I no longer knew what I wanted and wasn't sure if I could do it.

These thoughts, it turns out, are not uncommon among new parents facing such a diagnosis for their child.[10] Based on interviews with hundreds of women, anthropologist Rayna Rapp reports that "many mothers of newborns with Down syndrome recalled praying that their babies would die."[11] This "fleeting death wish" suggests just how extreme that sense of crisis feels, a turning point darkened by intense uncertainty. During that liminal period of not knowing, waiting for the dice to settle, Tiffani and I plodded toward the threshold of a new world, fearful of the change ahead.

Near the end of the week, the pediatrician called us at home in the evening. She asked if we could see her in the morning. Of course, I said. And then I spent one more sleepless night by myself on the sofa, hoping. Just hoping. In retrospect, this was absurd. If it had been "good news," she would have told us over the phone. But I allowed myself to languish in denial for one more night, to ignore a reality I already knew to be true.

We arrived at the doctor's office the next morning and were quickly greeted by the pediatrician. She was dressed casually in jeans; it was clearly not a typical day in the office. She had come in on her day off just to deliver the diagnosis. She ushered us into a consultation room and closed the door behind her. Children's books and magazines lined a rack on the wall, and some toys lay on the ground in the corner, just behind the examination table. Red, blue, yellow, and green beads hung from a maze of rigid wires fixed to a wooden base. Would Michaela someday play with those toys, I wondered?

"There's no easy way to say this," she started. "I'm so sorry."

I was stunned, shocked into silence, even though it confirmed a truth I already knew, and I immediately felt like I was mourning someone's death. She handed us a book called *Babies with Down Syndrome: A New Parent's Guide*, packed with all sorts of information, courtesy of the state advocacy group Down Syndrome Association of Wisconsin. Among other essays, it includes a short piece called "Welcome to Holland," written in 1987 by Emily Perl Kingsley. It's a parable about ending up in a place you didn't expect to be and finding joy anyway. The pediatrician tried to summarize it and strongly suggested we read it. In that moment, the gesture felt trivializing and in the days that followed I avoided it out of protest. It would be five years before I came across it again and finally read it.

"I know this is not what you expected," she said as we prepared to leave. "And it's not your fault."

Tiffani had tears in her eyes.

"Oh, I know," continued the pediatrician. "You did all the right things. You read all the books. You ate the right food. You exercised. It's unfair, but it's nothing you did."

The pediatrician knew there would be struggles ahead, but also that things could have been worse. "I've had several Downs kiddos over the years, and I'll say one thing: They're such happy people. They really are."

They. Them. *Those people*, I thought. I looked over at Michaela and I didn't see my daughter anymore. I saw a "Downs baby."

I felt an urge to escape. I excused myself as Tiffani and Michaela waited for something in the doctor's office. I went for a walk to nowhere in particular, circling the hospital. Even though it was early March, still winter in Wisconsin, the sun was bright, and the temperature felt warm. Spring was just around the corner. I went to my car and put the keys in the ignition. I could leave, I thought. Just go. Drive.

Instead, I called my older brother. And cried.

I'm not sure at what point in my life I decided to pursue anthropology. I grew up largely in the Chicago suburbs and my high school years unfolded against the backdrop of strip malls and an upper middle-class neighborhood called Brook Hills, the kind of prefabricated place where the same handful of model homes repeat endlessly with minor alterations in brick or trim color. Manicured lawns and landscaping, swimming pools, and luxury cars functioned symbolically as showy claims to success, to having achieved the so-called American Dream. There was something empty about it all.

As a teenager, I was an unmotivated student, showing few signs of a potential scholar. As I entered my senior year of high school, my guidance counselor suggested I consider "a trade," something practical. I responded that my mom told me I had to go to college. Months later, I was lying on the couch with my girlfriend when I got a call from the athletic director at Trinity Christian College, a nearby conservative Christian college, who recruited me to play soccer. So that's what I did for three years, with one year at a community college. I changed majors several times and eventually settled on sociology, an area of study that sparked my intellectual curiosity and academic promise in a new way. I also befriended a group of rebellious, creative people, misfits who seemed out of place at that small, suburban campus. We took cross-country road trips, read books, and talked late into the night at a Greek diner, ordering nothing but coffee. I think that was the first time I heard of anthropology. One friend told me she wanted to become an anthropologist, to travel and explore the world, like a contemporary Margaret Mead. I was smitten.

Just as Mead did for Erik Erikson, my brother Jim has served as a strong, guiding presence in my life. He is a mere fifteen months older than me, and we have always had a reliable, supportive relationship, even during our more antagonistic adolescent years. When I called Jim from the hospital parking lot, he was in a skyscraper in downtown Chicago, pitching an advertising campaign to corporate executives. Jim is a successful art director and finds creative ways to manipulate consumer behavior. At first glance, his professional world seems incompatible with the discipline of anthropology, a scholarly field that in recent decades has fancied itself as an agent of progressive societal change and human betterment. But the type of cultural analysis that occurs in marketing and advertising resonates in striking ways with anthropology, and we have often bonded over our shared assessments of human behavior and society, of the class dynamics and racial fears that animate the suburban lifestyle we experienced growing up—he is just paid a lot more to think about and influence human behavior than I will ever be as a college professor. He left the meeting to talk with me, looking out a window as people busily moved about on the sidewalk below, some walking along the Chicago River toward the historic Wrigley Building and the grandiose Trump Tower. Sensing the panicked despair in my voice, he was utterly calm.

"Where are you?" he asked.

"I'm in my car, in the hospital parking lot," I responded, sobbing.

"Where's Tiffani?"

"She's still inside with Michaela. She has, she has . . ."

I struggled to say the words, to name it.

"She has Down syndrome," I finally whispered, even though I was alone in my car. After a long pause to catch my breath, I continued. "I just want to leave. I want to start driving and just keep going."

The text message I had sent him days earlier had given him time to prepare. He had researched Down syndrome and spoken with a colleague who had a child with Down syndrome. Much more than I had done in my state of denial.

"Yes, it'll be different," he said, "but it will be fine. Michaela will go to school. You'll coach her soccer team. She'll be a great cousin and sibling, and Aidric will be a better person for being a brother to her."

I hadn't thought of anything positive coming from this and was speechless. I listened in silence, head spinning with thoughts of what might or might not happen in the future.

"She has a family that loves her," he said. He was referring to me, to us.

I said nothing.

"We're planning to come up tomorrow," he continued, pausing for a moment. "I'll hop in my car and drive up right now, if you want."

"No," I responded. "That's not necessary." I imagined him walking to his car in the parking garage under Grant Park, leaving a bunch of corporate suits behind in a conference room, wondering what had happened to him. His confidence reassured me.

"Go take care of your family," he said. I turned the car off and went back in.

A year later Jim would be the one calling me, just before he admitted himself to a psychiatric ward at a hospital, losing his grip on reality. The paralyzing anxiety and undiagnosed obsessive compulsive disorder that he had first talked with me about several years prior would finally overwhelm him. But for now, he was helping me to confront my deepest fears, bringing me back from the brink.

I've since learned the urge to escape is common among parents who face a Down syndrome diagnosis.[12] The desire to run away expresses the emotional upheaval triggered by news that upends one's life script—the unconscious narrative of how life is supposed to unfold. Such a diagnosis is extremely disorienting.

Tiffani and I spent the day driving around and talking about how Down syndrome would change our lives. We pondered our future. Would Michaela ever be able to ride a bike? Would she learn to drive a car? What about college? Would she get married one day, or ever live on her own? We ended up having brunch at a trendy restaurant in downtown Eau Claire. I ordered eggs and wondered for the first time if people noticed that my baby was different. I felt out of place. I could barely look the server in the eyes as I asked for more coffee.

At the end of the day, I called my mom. I hadn't told my parents of our suspicions, and they had since returned to the Chicago suburbs from their brief initial visit after Michaela's birth. But it was time. Time to face what was in front us and take a step forward.

"Mom," I said, my voice cracking. She knew something was wrong and waited in silence. My breathing deepened. "Michaela has been diagnosed with Down syndrome."

I could still barely say it, but it came out more smoothly than when I'd first tried to tell Jim. I'm not sure how I expected my mom to respond, but she floored me, and initially left me bitter.

"So what?" she said, almost dismissively.

"Mom, what do you mean?"

"So what? What's the big deal?"

I felt like I was confronting a life-changing crisis and my mother didn't appear to give a shit, or at least failed to acknowledge the gravity of the situation. I know now that she was merely trying to convey that Down syndrome doesn't have to be perceived as exceptional or out of the ordinary.

"Ok, well," I said curtly, "please let Dad know. I got to go."

I was on my way to pick up Aidric from daycare and used that as an excuse to quickly end the call before she could say much else. I didn't really give her a chance to elaborate.

.   .   .   .   .

During that week, that period from birth to diagnosis, the foundation of my worldview, a belief system informed by my training in cultural anthropology, began to shift under my feet. Here I was, an expert in a discipline that studies and celebrates the diversity of humankind, struggling to come to terms with a child born different.

Part of what drew me to anthropology was fascination with other cultures. But there was also a sense of feeling unsettled about where I had come from. During my senior year of college as I researched the possibility of graduate school, I was attracted to the romantic notion of fieldwork in a foreign place. Having grown up in the Chicago suburbs, a setting I had come to view cynically as artificial and infatuated with sameness, I longed to encounter the strange and exotic. One day an English professor lent me a copy of *The Interpretation of Culture* by Clifford Geertz, and the playful, adventurous spirit conveyed in Geertz's writing—and his exploration of the symbolic systems that lend meaning to human experience—cemented my interest in cultural anthropology. Coursework in graduate school helped me to question my assumptions about cultural difference and the underlying beliefs that shaped my perceptions of self and other. Fieldwork promised the adventure of exploring other cultural worlds, learning new languages, seeing things from a new perspective. When Mead went to Samoa in the 1920s, it wasn't just for adventure. The journey also had pragmatic purposes. The idea of going to the field, of immersing oneself in another cultural setting, of experiencing a different world firsthand, was taking shape as a core method of anthropology, and has since become a rite of passage in the discipline. To become an anthropologist, you must *do anthropology*, and that typically means fieldwork. I studied Spanish in Oaxaca, and pursued fieldwork in Central America, living first in El Salvador and then in Costa Rica, and traveled throughout the region. These experiences helped shape me, helped deepen my appreciation for the varied ways to be human.

During graduate school, I learned that the Boasian legacy of cultural relativism and tolerance of diversity is sacrosanct. The seminar room in the Anthropology Department at Binghamton University, where I completed my degrees, is called the Boas Room. The image of Margaret Mead still holds an iconic place in the discipline's collective self-identity, even as scholars comb through the nuances and contradictions of her legacy. Beyond anthropology, Mead and her fellow Boasian contemporaries are today sometimes remembered as "renegades" who challenged the assumptions of scientific racism and preached a radical openness to appreciating human diversity during the Jim Crow era of racial apartheid in the United States and when Nazism surged and culminated with the Holocaust in Germany.[13] And, no doubt, we should celebrate their contributions.

But Mead also helped condemn Neil Erikson, someone like my daughter, to an abject life in an institution. When Neil's father called her, Mead was personally confronted with a situation that stretched the boundaries of what it means to be human. She could have counseled empathy, acceptance, and openness to the unexpected. She could have said, "So what?" But she didn't. She conformed to a dominant culture that segregated some people so far beyond of the bounds of normalcy that it seemed logical to remove a newborn from his unknowing mother. The weight of her culture was too much.

And the anthropological tradition she forged, that partly shaped me, also failed to live up to expectations. Just as Margaret Mead had recommended Neil be abandoned to an institution in 1944, a type of social death that left his siblings behind to mourn the loss of an infant brother, I found myself rejecting a newborn baby in 2015. Only it was my own.

Today, I am ashamed that I ever felt that way and I am grateful for the support system that tempered those initial feelings of rejection and urged me to imagine an ordinary future. My love for Michaela is so powerful that I can't fathom life without her. Yet, like other parents of children with disabilities, I initially reacted to Michaela's diagnosis as a profound rupture to my personal identity, in addition to my relationship with the field of anthropology.[14] Why was I initially devastated by her Down syndrome diagnosis? Why did I feel an impulse to reject her very humanity, despite my training as an anthropologist?

When we embrace the unfamiliar and the unexpected, we welcome the possibility of becoming something new. Like Mead, I was drawn to anthropology by the allure of studying other cultures. Mead, of course, also pioneered the move toward turning the anthropological perspective on oneself, looking at one's own culture as something strange. Anthropology is really about coming home and seeing things you once took for granted in a different light.

2 Features

"I'm sorry."

There were those words again. An expression of sorrow. Regret. Remorse. This time it was an administrator at my university—technically, my boss. The call surprised me. I didn't even know she had my cell phone number, much less that news of Michaela's birth had gotten to her so quickly. A day or two had passed since the diagnosis. Tiffani and I had told our close family and then I had anguished over how to share the news with my friends and colleagues. And then Tiffani posted this on social media:

> If I were not to post the following several sentences, you very likely would not ever guess that anything was going on . . . So, as impersonal as it may seem to give such an important "announcement" over Facebook, it saves me the difficult task of having to do it dozens of times when you meet my little sweetheart of a daughter. It was officially confirmed that Michaela has one little extra chromosome, landing her at a grand 47 rather than 46. For those who may not immediately understand the implications of such a thing, the result is a confirmed diagnosis of trisomy 21, aka Down syndrome. The world did not cease to spin, but the universe shifted around me and my family. Whether it is true or not, nearly everything seems different at one level or another. Expectations I didn't realize I had/have came to the fore and nearly crushed all the joy out of having a new baby. To say that it is difficult

very honest

18

to articulate my new world view is an understatement of grand proportion. Genetics and statistics. Two of the most fascinating and devastating topics in my current and future reality. Though the risk is somewhere between 1:700 to 1:1000, depending on what reports/studies you read, learning that your child is in fact that one, it doesn't matter how large the number on the other side of the ratio might be . . . one is all that matters. We are adjusting to the idea as well as could be expected, and look forward to our joyful, albeit somewhat different than anticipated, journey ahead.

I could not have said it better and was relieved when she posted the statement. It expressed many of the feelings I also was grappling with, and it marked a sort of public recognition that allowed for taking a step forward. For the most part, it spared us having to share the news repeatedly and manage people's awkward responses. But some still felt a need to reach out in more personal terms.

I was at a trendy coffee shop called the Raw Deal when my cell phone rang. The coffee shop occupies a restored historic building, a former general store that opened in the early twentieth century when Menomonie was still known as a lumber town. Natural light floods the cavernous café through front and side windows, reflecting off the tin ceiling. A second-level loft looks down over the space. As you walk in, the acrid smell of roasting coffee beans greets you, the heavy smoke vented to the outside. You can smell it from blocks away. I was seated at a large, wooden high-top table, drinking beer, which is served by most coffee shops in western Wisconsin. The administrator had never called me before.

"I have a sense of what you're feeling right now," she said. "I know there is nothing I can really say except, I'm sorry. I'm sorry."

I knew that she still provided care for an adult child with a cognitive disability. That she called me was a touching gesture, one parent reaching out to another. She was greeting me as a newcomer in a foreign land understood only by other inhabitants, like a native Samoan welcoming Margaret Mead upon her arrival. It is a connection that has shaped our professional relationship and friendship in the years since, and I cherish it.

Like the doctor who delivered the diagnosis, however, she was also unwittingly suggesting how I should channel my own feelings and reactions: grief. Unlike in other momentous occasions in life, there is no cultural script for how to support a loved one whose child is diagnosed with

Down syndrome or other conditions widely perceived as undesirable. My initial sense of loss was reinforced by well-meaning friends and family. While some offered support in a positive way that avoided casting judgement, others expressed sympathy, echoing the doctor who had delivered the diagnosis. Seemingly kind words or careful avoidance sent an unspoken message. *Grieve a tragic event and envision a difficult journey.*

"Thank you," I responded. "I appreciate your support."

I didn't know what else to say.

As I ended the call, however, I was feeling profoundly ambivalent. Michaela's diagnosis had overturned my world. I was deep in the process of coming to terms with it. Those around me were cuing up grief as the proper emotional response, offering a framework through which to understand my experience and perceive my daughter anew. But I found these gestures and frameworks unsatisfying. What were they sorry for anyway? Sorry that my child was not "perfect"? Sorry that we had the "wrong" baby?

The next day, another administrator called, another supervisor who had never called me at home before, reaching out in an awkward gesture of support, like a guest at a surprise birthday party for someone who does not wish to celebrate the inevitable passage of time. I was standing in the kitchen of our house, floors uneven from a century of use, generations of families before us, wood trim painted white, the plaster walls a milky green avocado color. I looked out at fresh snow glistening in the backyard.

"Conditions have improved so much for handicapped kids," they said.

The somewhat antiquated language caught my attention and struck me as an odd way to describe an infant. I thought of my great-grandfather adjusting his hearing aid. I recalled how he shuffled with the support of his metal folding walker into the bathroom, or how he gripped the car door with unsteady hands as he attempted to lift himself up and out of the car and into his wheelchair. I thought of handicapped parking spots, of attempting to push my grandfather up steep ramps or over curbs, of the times my brother and I as children played in his wheelchair or climbed on his walker for fun. I had always assumed disability was the plight of the elderly, a mere inconvenience to the young and able.

Was my daughter handicapped?

Not long after, a close friend inquired about my "special needs" baby, a phrase that stung and bewildered me. Michaela had not had any health problems or unique issues, and other than the diagnosis, caring for Michaela as a baby was uneventful. The infant stage is a predictable cycle of eating, sleeping, and diapering, of meeting all the basic needs of a creature entirely dependent on others for its very existence, a state of vulnerability that all humans experience when they first enter the world. In fact, people experience this mutual interdependency throughout most of their life. We are never really, truly self-reliant. What baby, I thought, doesn't have special needs?

I would soon come to realize that expressions of pity are often subtle, often indirect or with unintentional impact, sometimes masquerading as support—codewords that disguise a sense of disappointment, tinged with stigma. They carry the weight of history, unspoken prejudice setting boundaries around taken-for-granted categories of normalcy.

.   .   .   .   .

Though they share that extra chromosome, Neil Erikson and my daughter Michaela were born into very different worlds. The condition now known as Down syndrome was first described by the medical doctor John Langdon Down in the late 1860s, when he was superintendent of the Earlswood Asylum for Idiots, a Victorian-era institution in England. The phrase *idiot asylum* sounds foreign to modern ears, but as a concept, "idiocy" took shape during the Enlightenment to describe individuals unable to manage their own affairs, requiring the care of the state. As Western conceptions of personhood and citizenship came to emphasize rational decision-making and notions of a unified, self-reliant individual, idiocy marked an opposite. By Down's time, related terms such as "feebleminded" and "imbecile" were being used as diagnostic categories distinct from "insanity" or the merely destitute, which were understood as temporary or occasional episodes. This fostered efforts to remove so-called feebleminded children from poorhouses or asylums housing adults. Down later opened his own private institution, called the Normansfield Training Institution for Imbeciles, which was operated by his sons after his death in 1896. While superintendent at Earlswood, Down observed a pattern of

all very painful

physical features among some of the children under his care, such as slight stature, a "flat and broad" face, "roundish" cheeks, "obliquely placed" eyes, a small nose, and what he perceived as a long tongue.[1] He interpreted this pattern in terms of the dominant racial typologies circulating at the time and classified the children as "Mongols."

Such typologies have roots even earlier than Down's lifetime. In 1775, Johann Blumenbach's influential *On the Natural Variety of Humankind* formalized some of the categories being used in Western society to divide human populations based on geography and visible physical features. He coined the label "Caucasian" to encompass the peoples of Europe. Four other categories were already in use: "Ethiopians" for the peoples of Africa; "Americans" for people native to the Americas; "Mongolians" for the peoples of Asia; and "Malay" for the peoples of the Pacific. Blumenbach thought that all human populations could be traced to a single origin, the Caucasian, which over time had degenerated due to environmental factors, such as poor diet or continual exposure to extreme temperatures.[2] "For Blumenbach," explains historian Charles King, "Caucasians were the ur-source from which all subsequent varieties of humans had devolved."[3] When Down gazed at a group of his inmates at Earlswood who all looked similar, he thought he saw a variant of Mongolians.

Down fancied himself something of an anthropologist, a term used broadly at the time to describe intellectual explorers of human origins and variation. While trained as a medical doctor, Down was also engaged in debates about the evolution of humankind. In 1859, Darwin's *On the Origin of Species* described the biological process of natural selection and proposed a theory of common descent to account for the evolution of life on earth. Darwin's later work turned to the evolutionary development of humans, asserting that all humans share a common biological origin. But Darwin lacked the fossil evidence to show an evolutionary link between humans and other primates. In *The Descent of Man,* first published in 1871, he suggested that both "idiots" and "savages" could be studied as the living evidence of this missing link, and he compared these "least developed human beings" to the "most highly evolved animals."[4]

Down followed these debates closely, attending seminars and lecturing at the London Anthropological Society in the 1860s. The emerging field of anthropology was largely preoccupied with how to classify physical variation among humans, and many early anthropologists speculated on the fixed "ethnic" or "racial" divisions of humanity, viewed through a lens of racial hierarchy. They fiercely debated whether what they perceived as distinct races shared an evolutionary starting point or represented separate species entirely. Many scientists (and others claiming to be experts) obsessed over how to measure the physical proportions of the human body and then define categories of humans based on these measurements, a practice eventually known as anthropometry. Skulls, and thus brains, were of special interest, and craniometry—measuring the part of the skull that holds the brain—fueled wild generalizations about the supposedly innate mental capacities or temperaments of entire groups of people.

In the United States, race dominated scientific inquiry, with anthropologists and others studying features of the body to demonstrate the supposedly innate inferiority of people of African descent. This effort sought first to justify slavery, then to reinforce a racial caste system of white supremacy following the Civil War, relying heavily on assumptions about idiocy and disability. After moving to the United States in the 1850s, for instance, the Swiss naturalist Louis Agassiz became a prominent creationist and supporter of polygeny, or the idea that different races had separate origins. He promoted a "scientific" explanation of races as separate from one another and hierarchically ranked, describing non-White peoples as physically and mentally deficient. He warned that the mixing of races threatened to "impair" the dominance of Caucasians.[5] Similarly mobilizing science in support of racial prejudice, Samuel George Morton promoted polygeny and amassed a significant collection of skulls as his empirical evidence. His flawed measurements, presented in publications such as his 1839 *Crania Americana*, were embraced as "objective" descriptions of racial difference and Caucasians' innate intellectual advantages. In the 1860s, scientists such as Paul Broca sought to demonstrate the biological inferiority of non-White peoples, measuring brains to advance arguments about innate intelligence.[6] Black people were often described as having defective bodies and minds, as being naturally feebleminded, as lacking the full capacity for reason. The physician Samuel Cartwright, for example, maintained that enslaved Black people were physically deficient and prone to "diseases of the mind" that caused them to flee their captors.[7] If White people embodied ability and proficiency, the physical and mental capacity for full citizenship, Black people were portrayed through images of deficiency, impairment, and disease—the language of disability.[8]

In his 1867 article "Observations on an Ethnic Classification of Idiots," Down sought to contribute to scientific discussions of human variation, while adding to a nascent taxonomy of idiocy. He was stunned by the physical resemblance shared by some inmates in his asylum. You would think they were "born to the same family," he wrote.[9] According to medical historian Owen Conor Ward, "the basis of his ethnic classification was the measurement of the diameters of the head and the identification of specific facial features from photographs which he took himself." It's well established that Down was an avid photographer and sought to document visible characteristics, the raw evidence of types.[10] Down even corresponded with Darwin in 1873 about the ear of a four-year-old "microcephalic idiot" who had died under his supervision. He sent Darwin a photograph of the ear before dissecting it.[11] Studying such photographs, Down perceived an "ethnic" resemblance to a more "primitive" racial type among some of his inmates.

To explain the birth of Mongol children from Caucasian parents, he invoked a version of recapitulation theory that supported the assertion of racial reversion or degeneration. Theories of recapitulation were not uncommon during this period.[12] The nineteenth-century German naturalist Ernst Haeckel, for instance, asserted that "the embryo of an advanced form of life (such as the human) retraces, or recapitulates, the phases in the evolutionary history of its race" during its development.[13] Even Darwin suggested that idiots could be looked at, in his words, as "a case of reversion" to earlier stages of human evolution, "arrested in development" and displaying characteristics of a "lower animal type."[14]

Many scientists of the period drew on recapitulation theory to justify racial, gender, and class hierarchies. As science historian Stephen Jay Gould explains, some suggested that "the *adults* of *inferior* groups must be like *children* of *superior* groups, for the child represents a primitive adult ancestor. If adult blacks and women are like white male children, then they are living representatives of an ancestral stage in the evolution of white males. An anatomical theory for ranking races—based on entire bodies, not only on heads—had been found."[15] Following this line of thinking, the "criminal anthropologist" Cesare Lombroso claimed to be able to identify "natural-born criminals" based on physical features or stigmata.[16] Key to his approach was the notion that criminality is an evolutionary throwback to so-called primitive humanity—the stigmata of criminality were "apish" in nature. Lombroso and other criminal anthropologists of his time also asserted a link between disability and criminality, associating the latter with epilepsy, insanity, and mental deficiency. Lombroso's physical stigmata and their association with disabling conditions were equated with "moral degeneration."

In this intellectual context, the dawning of anthropology as a modern discipline, Down offered a theory of racial reversion to explain what he called the Mongol features of his White English patients. For some reason, his group of White inmates had reverted in utero to a more primitive ethnic or racial state, falling many steps down the evolutionary ladder. This aligned Down with monogenism, and he concluded that his observations, in his words, supported "arguments in favour of the unity of the human species," a progressive position for his period.[17] At the same time, he helped strengthen the association of disability with animality, with the nonhuman. A boundary had been drawn. He also furthered racist thinking that marked, as Gould puts it, "undesirable whites as biological representatives of [racially] lower groups," reinforcing the perception of non-White peoples as innately feebleminded and morally suspect.[18] From Darwin to Down, notions of intellectual disability and racial difference were interwoven, an evolutionary association with animality marking certain groups as outside the parameters of the human.[19]

. . . . . .

John Langdon Down's description of a "Mongolian type of idiocy" resulting from racial "degeneration," just a few paragraphs in a scant three-page paper, remained a small contribution in his time. He even complained to Darwin that his paper "did not excite much interest."[20] The explanation was largely ignored in the United States, where people of African descent were already viewed as the bottom of a racial hierarchy. One physician soon documented "negro mongoloid idiots," which from an American perspective could not be explained by recapitulation or racial reversion.[21] Nevertheless, terms such as "mongolism" or "mongoloid" found their way into medical terminology in the late nineteenth century, persisting well into the twentieth.[22] The mongoloid became a diagnostic category and a type.

The category gained meaning in relation to the development of institutions that not only provided care for people, but also "defined normative and deviant bodies and minds," as historian Kim Nielsen writes, demarcating spaces where the undesirable would be sent.[23] As urban industrial development unfolded in Europe and the United States, private groups and governments began to invest in institutions to care for "feebleminded" children separate from asylums for "chronically insane" adults. Homes for the feebleminded were created with a charitable vision, often drawing on the thinking of figures such as Edouard Séguin, who in 1839 founded in Paris one of the first such schools under the premise that idiots, imbeciles, and the feebleminded could be educated. In the United States in the late nineteenth and early twentieth centuries, such institutions were commonly established as "colonies" in remote locations where an innocent class of people would be "trained" as productive members of a modern, capitalist society, emphasizing tasks like farming, basket-weaving, or operating machinery. Disability was being associated with lack of economic productivity, so the goal was to cultivate workers who could contribute.

By the 1890s, however, the existence of these institutions intersected with the rise of scientific eugenics, and "homes" or "colonies" for the feebleminded became increasingly segregated from society, a place to hide the "unfit." Their function shifted from education to confinement. The eugenics movement also breathed new life into the dehumanizing racial connotations associated with the diagnosis of mongolism.

The term eugenics was first developed by Francis Galton in 1883 to refer to "the science of improving the stock" of physical, mental, and behavioral traits supposedly inherited by a population or passed down from generation to generation.[24] What were perceived as "beneficial" or desirable traits could be promoted in the population, while harmful or undesirable ones could be discouraged and eventually eliminated through proper breeding. Eugenics, of course, was always infused with racist and ethnocentric attitudes—with proponents assuming their way of life was inherently the best. People with economic and political power, most often

White, viewed themselves as naturally superior, as representing the peak of human evolution. "Intermixing" with non-White peoples was commonly perceived as damaging to so-called civilized society. The association between race and mental deficiency made by figures such as Agassiz, Morton, and Cartwright—and Darwin's and Down's assumption that so-called idiocy represented a more "primitive" evolutionary state—meant that categories of undesirable people were viewed not only through a racial lens, but also in terms of impairment and disability.[25]

As an intellectual field, eugenics developed hand in hand with the formation of new branches of knowledge such as statistics. Galton was "a pioneer of modern statistics" and drew an explicit connection between measuring the boundaries of normalcy and the quest to improve humans.[26] The very notion that populations have measurable "norms" gave rise to inverse categories of "abnormality," identifying people who were perceived to deviate from the newly imagined average.[27] Deviations from the statistical norm were associated with perceived "traits," taken as innate and measurable, assumed to define entire groups. Those traits deemed undesirable came to mark groups that eugenicists saw as "unfit" for reproduction. For example, in 1911, Karl Pearson, a leading eugenics thinker and the head of the Applied Statistics Department at University College in London, defined the unfit as "the habitual criminal, the professional tramp, the tuberculous, the insane, the mentally defective, the alcoholic, the diseased from birth or from excess."[28] Nineteenth-century terms such as feebleminded, used broadly to describe people with various cognitive conditions, were reinscribed as "mentally defective" or "abnormal." In the context of early twentieth-century efforts to foster social welfare and public health, the mentally defective were increasingly viewed as a "menace" to society—a threat to national fitness and a burden on the state.[29]

Building from the previous century's focus on anthropometry and craniometry, in the early twentieth century scientists sought to measure the internal capacities of the mind. In 1904, the French psychological researcher Alfred Binet developed techniques to evaluate children's reasoning skills and analytical abilities, what became known as intelligence testing. His initial vision was to identify students who struggled in mainstream educational systems, then to find alternatives to help them learn.[30] He cautioned against using his techniques to try to rank children or identify innate characteristics that would somehow define their potential. He saw his techniques, and statistical tools such as an intelligence scale, as a resource for enhancing potential and reforming flawed education systems that focused on rote learning. The tests were used in the French school system and refined with physician Theodore Simon. What became known as the Binet-Simon Scale presumed to measure a child's "mental age," as distinct from chronological age, and became a basis for determining an "intelligence quotient" or IQ.

When the techniques were taken up by scientists in the United States, however, they were tethered to a "hereditarian theory of IQ," and to the eugenic assumption that they measured innate qualities passed along from one generation to the next.[31] Henry H. Goddard, the director of research at the Vineland Training School for Feeble-Minded Girls and Boys in New Jersey, was one of the first to bring the Binet-Simon scale to the United States. He used it to invent the "moron." Like Down in the previous century, Goddard wanted to advance a taxonomy of the feebleminded children under his supervision. The terms "idiot" and "imbecile" were in common usage, with "imbeciles" slightly more capable than "idiots." "Feebleminded" was bit more ambiguous, sometimes working as a generic catch-all phrase, sometimes used in reference to those deemed more capable of learning than idiots and imbeciles. Goddard coined the word "morons," inspired by a Greek word for foolish, for those trainable "high-grade defectives."[32] He maintained that intelligence was a unitary thing that described a basic human capacity with variations across groups. Some groups were endowed with great advantage, others destined to failure. Racism, sexism, and class exploitation were thus conveniently blamed on biology. The masses of uneducated workers toiling away under the precarious conditions of early industrial capitalism must be responsible for their own poverty and misery—they were morons of "defective stock."[33]

Drawing on themes circulating since at least the mid-nineteenth century, he also asserted a link between mental deficiency and immoral behaviors ranging from alcoholism and criminality to sexual promiscuity. The feebleminded were a menace to society, and they liked to sleep around, breeding uncontrollably. In 1912, Goddard published *The Kallikak Family*, a book that purported to examine the family history of a feebleminded girl enrolled at his school.[34] It told the story of "Deborah Kallikak" (whose real name was Emma Wolverton), a resident classified as a "high-grade moron." Goddard claimed to have researched her family tree and found that she descended from a successful Revolutionary War officer who had gallantly sired offspring with his legal spouse and then ignobly seeded another line of descendants with a "mentally defective" barmaid. In contrast to the legitimate descendants, who all formed part of a successful New England family composed of doctors, lawyers, and ministers, the barmaid's lineage faired much worse, with hundreds of descendants found to be "sexually immoral," alcoholics, epileptics, or criminals. Deborah, of course, represented the barmaid's family lineage. *The Kallikak Family* was immensely popular, offering a tragic story of what happens when morons are left to their own devices: they set into motion great social and economic burdens on society, which snowball over the generations.[35]

Under the guise of science, such books sought to articulate the types of bodies and minds that supposedly constitute ideal citizens, positioning the undesirable as a danger to society. While Goddard saw the feebleminded as a reproductive threat from within the populace, he also feared that immigrants presented an external one. In possibly the first use of systematic intelligence testing in the United States, Goddard oversaw studies that screened immigrants arriving at Ellis Island. He trained observers to visually identify the potentially feebleminded, presumably based on physical characteristics (a look, a demeanor, *something* about them), and then pull them aside for testing. Goddard "discovered" that immigrants from Southern and Eastern Europe, groups already facing prejudice and discrimination in the United States, were often morons. Stephen Jay Gould asks us to imagine the following scenario in the context of 1913: vulnerable people endure an oceanic voyage in steerage, and they're tired, hungry, and scared; they are fleeing poverty, violence, or political persecution; they speak little English; they've probably never gone to school or even had reason to hold a pencil before. They're suddenly plucked from a line. Then they're briefly shown a visual image and asked to draw it from memory, or given other images with missing parts to fill in, or presented with other tasks that supposedly measure innate intelligence. Of course, they perform poorly.[36]

Intelligence testing was promoted nationally in the United States at a time when the expansion of compulsory elementary education had "brought millions of children under the surveillance of the state," creating a new administrative urgency to gather statistical information about the character of populations.[37] Intelligence scales were used to differentiate between supposedly normal and abnormal children, and increasingly "to identify and segregate the mentally unfit."[38] Large-scale assessment was supercharged by the use of intelligence testing in military recruitment during World War I, a program pushed by scientists such as Harvard psychologist Robert Yerkes. He saw testing recruits as an opportunity to generate lots of data, maintaining that intelligence testing would provide a more scientific, empirical basis for psychological research.[39] Like the tests at Ellis Island, the Army Mental Tests were systematically flawed, but the results were nevertheless taken as objective—and they revealed an alarming degree of "below average" intelligence among certain groups, particularly Black people, as well as recent immigrants from Southern and Eastern Europe. Many conscripts came from poverty, lacked English language proficiency, or were illiterate. Their performance on tests was heavily influenced by questionable testing conditions and other factors such as socioeconomic background, linguistic skills, literacy, and cultural knowledge. But the Army Mental Tests generated large amounts of statistical information that was accepted by many as providing insight into the inherent qualities of different groups, and the results would impact policymaking for decades.

The data was used by policymakers to justify racial segregation and propose new limits on immigration. New versions of intelligence testing were developed, such as the Stanford-Binet Scale, which sought to rank IQ based on a statistically derived distribution curve, propelling into the twentieth-century popular imagination the notion that intelligence is singular, innate, and hierarchical—and that there is such thing as an average or "normal" mind.

Early twentieth-century fears of the growing ranks of "mental defectives" were deeply racialized. Jim Crow laws protected the racial inequalities formed out of the ashes of plantation economies, while legal and policy initiatives sought to establish the terms of Whiteness—and thus belonging—as new waves of immigrants arrived from Europe. After World War I, eugenics increasingly informed government policy related to immigration, with many calling for quotas or restrictions on groups deemed undesirable due to innate features. Books such as Madison Grant's *The Passing of the Great Race*, first published in 1916, inspired a generation of racial science and policymaking, purporting to show that humans could be cleanly divided into racial categories.[40] Grant argued, playing to White anxieties at the time, that "advanced" or "superior" races were under threat of being "diluted" through mixture with "primitive" races. The "dilution" of the "great race" would produce a kind of reversion to so-called primitive racial states. Grant wrote that "the cross between a white man and an Indian is an Indian; the cross between a white man and a negro is a negro; the cross between a white man and a Hindu is a Hindu; and the cross between any of the three European races and a Jew is a Jew."[41]

It's out of this context that intellectual figures such as Margaret Mead took shape. Her mentor, Franz Boas, a wily, German-born scholar who had established himself in the anthropology department at Columbia University, challenged conventional thinking about human variation. He was a proponent of rigorous, empirical observation, but he also acknowledged that Western scientists were products of their own cultures, and that their views of the world would inevitably reflect underlying, unspoken beliefs and values. This doesn't, he argued, disqualify the claims of scientists, but means they need to examine their assumptions. He questioned what others took for granted as obvious or part of the natural order of things, particularly claims about racial difference.

Boas participated in government-funded studies of the physical characteristics of Italians, Jews, and other immigrant groups from Eastern, Central, and Southern Europe, but drew very different conclusions than figures such as Goddard or Grant.[42] He concluded in 1911 that considerable physical variation exists within presumed racial groups, and that the physical features of groups change from generation to generation depending on social and environmental conditions. Human biology is much more malleable than had been previously thought, he argued. Boas questioned the idea of race as fixed and heritable, as reduceable to innate traits. Much of what was chalked up to human instinct could be better explained as learned cultural behavior. "To speak of hereditary characteristics of a human race as a whole has no meaning," Boas argued in a critique of Grant's book on racial dilution.[43] Boas disputed the claims and methods of eugenics in countless reviews and essays, culminating in his 1929 book *Anthropology and Modern Life*. His views, however, and the evidence he amassed, were largely dismissed by policymakers at the time, and the restrictive, xenophobic Immigration Act of 1924 set quotas that favored immigrants from Northern and Western Europe, groups perceived as "Whiter" and of superior stock.

In many ways, the Boasian project became one of challenging the categories of thought that shaped the Western imagination, divisions and types assumed to be innate and universal. This was a project he handed off to his students, including Mead. While a student at Columbia in 1924, she conducted research on intelligence testing among Italian immigrants in New York City, administering tests to hundreds of children and comparing the results with how much English was spoken in their homes. This line of inquiry reflected a larger critique of intelligence testing. Critics argued that environmental conditions, not innate qualities, explained the results being reported by the Army Mental Tests and scientists such as Goddard. Based on her research, Mead argued that language, status, and other social conditions, including "the attitude of the subject toward the tests," affect scores. She found that if more English was spoken at home, children scored better—which suggests that sociocultural conditions influence performance on these tests. She raised these questions in her first published article, titled "The Methodology of Racial Testing." Intelligence testing didn't so much measure the "mental traits" of different groups, as it did the relative linguistic and cultural knowledge of test takers. When her article was published in the *American Journal of Sociology* in 1926, Mead was out of the country in Samoa, conducting the fieldwork that would rocket her to public fame. Based on her research in Samoa, she would argue that childhood and adolescence are experienced differently across cultures. Dimensions of human existence such as sexuality, assumed to be universal or innate, are profoundly shaped by culture.

The idea that something called culture shapes human behavior and potential—culture being a learned system of meanings and values, relative and arbitrary, created by people—was radical against the backdrop of eugenics. If qualities like intelligence or sexuality are not fixed and universal, then what is? Another of Boas's students, Ruth Benedict, pushed this critique beyond the discussion of racial types that so heavily dominated the era. Like Mead, Benedict probed how culture shapes psychological and emotional experience. But Benedict was also moderately deaf, a result of childhood measles. Her deafness was a partially disabling condition that likely shaped her relationship to conceptions of normality.[44] In her 1934 article "Anthropology and the Abnormal," Benedict asks to what extent categories of normal and abnormal are unique to their cultural settings. Abnormality was increasingly taken as diagnostic among medical scientists in the United States, indicative of some underlying anomaly consistent across humanity. But what if, Benedict argued, it simply reflects a culture's way of classifying certain behaviors that are valued by people in that culture, while marking out other behaviors that they've come to stigmatize or even demonize? If standards are culturally relative, what does it mean to classify someone as abnormal? She gave examples from non-Western cultures where people prone to seizures, schizophrenia, or manic depression aren't stigmatized as ill or mentally deficient, but instead are "socially placed" and even celebrated in roles such as shamans or trance seekers. She also gave the example of homosexuality, viewed in the 1930s as deviant, if not pathological, as a behavior sanctioned as normal in other cultures or even at other points in Western history. "The concept of the normal is properly a variant of the concept of the good," she wrote, recognizing that claims about normality are morally charged.

"It is that which society has approved."[45]

.   .   .   .   .

While Boas and his students questioned the very terms of the discussion, lines were being drawn in the United States to demarcate the boundaries of humanity and exclude the abnormal, and mongolism would fall into a category that even Mead failed to challenge in 1944 when Erikson called her with news of Neil's birth. Medical doctors and other commentators continued to shape a diagnosis that characterized mongolism as subhuman, and they fixated on physical features as evidence. Heads, eyes, necks, tongues, ears—all measured, photographed, dissected, and classified.

In 1908, Down's son, Reginald Langdon-Down, who by then managed the Normansfield institution founded by his late father, described a single crease running across the palm of some of his inmates diagnosed with mongolism. He named it a "simian crease," viewing it as an apish feature, like those described by Lombroso and others in the previous century. Reginald had a strong personal connection to mongolism, beyond the fact that his institution housed such children. In a remarkable twist of fate, given that his father had classified the condition, Reginald's only son, named Jonathan, was born in 1905 with mongolism.[46] A family photograph featuring Reginald includes Jonathan, who reportedly was a "well-loved member of the family, living a happy life to the ripe old age of 65."[47] Another photograph taken by Reginald captures Jonathan riding a bike. Jonathan attended a local school in his early years and his mother, Jane, "refused to admit that there was anything at all different about him."[48] When Jane died in 1917, Jonathan spent his days at Normansfield with a caretaker, and was only formally admitted there in 1951, when his father retired.[49]

Among the family papers is a sketch of the "simian crease," the drawing attributed to Reginald.[50] The sketch features a child's hand, palm facing upward, as if resting in a parent's lap. Over a century later, I find the image striking because I've looked at my own child's hand from this vantage point many times. Now and then, Michaela sits on my lap, her back against my chest. We'll be reading books or watching television. Her hair is thin and soft, and the back of her head nestles under my chin, against my neck. She pulls my arm snugly around her. I feel the rhythm of her heartbeat. I look over her shoulder at her hand resting on her leg. A mesh of lines run diagonally across her palm. As far as I can tell, Michaela does not have a noticeable single crease, but her pinky finger curves slightly inward, like the hand in Reginald's drawing. It's unknown whose hand is featured in the 1908 sketch, made just three years after Jonathan's birth. But I'd like to think Jonathan is sitting in his father's lap, while Reginald peers lovingly at his son's hand, contemplating the beautiful features of his child.

It's just as likely that Reginald was studying his son's physical features for other reasons. Reginald never publicly acknowledged Jonathan's condition, even as he reported on "Mongolian imbecility" at medical conferences and corresponded with parents who had sent their own children to

Normansfield.[51] He supported eugenics, testifying as an expert about the hereditarian nature of mongolism and "the relative threat that feeble-mindedness posed to society."[52] The term he coined, "simian crease," exemplified renewed fears of racial degeneracy. Although Reginald questioned the specific explanation of racial degeneration offered decades earlier by his father, in 1905, just months after Jonathan's birth, he speculated that, if anything, the condition "must be a reversion to a type even further back than the Mongol stock, from which some ethnologists believe all the various races of men have sprung."[53]

This passage found its way into *The Mongol in Our Midst*, a racist eugenic tract in which Francis Crookshank claimed that "Mongolian imbecility" represented a reversion to orangutans.[54] Crookshank was a British medical doctor with an interest in epidemiology and psychology, and a member of the Royal College of Physicians. *The Mongol in Our Midst* was first published in 1924 as a short book that was part of the "To-Day and To-Morrow" series, which brought the latest science to a popular audience. Crookshank drew on the extensive body of anthropometric research that sought to measure the physical features of diverse humans and categorize them into racial types. Framed as an objective, scientific review of existing research, his racist anthropological analysis revived the spirt of John Langdon Down's initial theory of racial atavism. But whereas for Down the appearance of "Mongolian" characteristics was evidence of the unity of humankind, Crookshank, who maintained that different human races descended from distinct species of apes, saw it as a dilution of the purity of the White race. Mongolian imbecility was the consequence of a perilous intermixing of races at some point in the evolutionary history of separate human species.[55]

The anthropologist and linguist Edward Sapir, who studied under Franz Boas at Columbia University, wrote a scathing critique of *The Mongol in Our Midst* in 1925, part of a review article titled "The Race Problem."[56] Sapir blasted the book as some sort of twisted joke, all the while recognizing it formed part of a flourishing genre of racial science. "The author's thesis," he wrote, "need only be stated to be refuted with a laugh." Sapir feared, though, that Crookshank (or some of his readers) believed the argument about racial degeneracy. "Our guess, however, would be that he is serious," continued Sapir. "Should it appear, in the wash, that Mr. Crookshank has been holding a huge chuckle in reserve, we should be the first to take off our hat to him as one of the most brilliant hoaxers in contemporary scientific literature."

In addition to physical features related to eyes, head shape, and lines in the palm, Crookshank argued that the supposed behavioral traits of Mongolian imbeciles (sitting cross-legged "like a Buddha" and stunted speech patterns) demonstrated their link to the "Mongolian race." Sapir dismissed this, but also attacked the logic employed by Crookshank, particularly the notion that behaviors or cultural phenomenon are transmitted biologically or could be explained through reference to human "genetics," a word only coined in 1905. Sapir criticized the "characteristic illusion of the biologist, who is persuaded into accepting his genetic technique as a sufficient interpretive guide to the cultural behavior of man."[57] In attacking this logic, Sapir was engaging the wider national discussion about race, as well as debates about human nature and nurture. Even authors who did not subscribe to eugenics commonly mistook learned behaviors to be biologically determined and tended to understand their own cultural beliefs as somehow natural or universal. Sapir, of course, following Boas, viewed behavior and culture as developing within their own very particular, historically shaped contexts.

Sapir called for explaining cultural phenomenon on their own terms and in their own settings—that is, as cultural phenomenon. Biologists, for instance, shouldn't be drawing conclusions about human behavior based on evidence drawn from human biology. "The cultural process is carried by human organisms, to be sure," wrote Sapir, a reference to the fact that humans are biological as well as cultural animals. But culture "is no more truly explainable in terms of biology than the ever-changing aspect of the wind-blown sea is explainable as a specific resultant of the chemistry of sea water."[58]

The Mongol in Our Midst embodied two powerful early twentieth-century eugenic imperatives, brought together in a shallow revival of Down's theory of racial reversion: anthropometrics and intelligence testing. It was never about the people defined as having this condition, or even the condition itself. "Mongolian imbecility" was merely a foil, a visible manifestation of "mental deficiency" used to express fears about the degeneracy of White racial supremacy. Even Sapir didn't question the subhuman status assigned to people categorized as Mongolian imbeciles, never acknowledging their humanity.

Though *The Mongol in Our Midst* drew mixed scientific reviews, it found success with a general audience that increasingly viewed immigration as a source of racial dilution, and difference within society itself as a threat to national fitness. After its initial publication as a pithy 123-page tract, the book was expanded in subsequent editions, published as a 500-page tomb in 1931. It was translated into German in 1928, forming part of an intellectual movement among the Nazis with devastating consequences. Sapir had mocked the book as a joke but recognized its alarming appeal. Why books like *The Mongol in Our Midst* are published as if they have scientific merit "would be hard to say, but it is undeniable that they are delightful interludes," he wrote, "in the grim and weary drama of race-discussion that we are in for these days."

.   .   .   .   .

After her diagnosis, Michaela's physical features suddenly took on new meaning for me, suddenly looked strange. In the week after she was born, we entered a world that threatened to strip her of her humanity and turn her into a diagnosis. Where I had initially seen my infant daughter, I now only saw Down syndrome. The diagnosis had become overdetermining, a thick lens through which I perceived my child's body and her future. I thought about Down syndrome every day. I was hyperconscious of the diagnosis. I looked over the photos taken when she was born. How did I not see it, I wondered? Hadn't it been obvious, even from the first moment? Coming to terms with the diagnosis was a process. For months, I would find myself thinking about Down syndrome all the time, noticing it in Michaela when I looked at her, looking for it in others.

Several months after her diagnosis, we happened to take Michaela and Aidric to the Minnesota State Fair. In the Chicago suburbs where I grew up, every summer a carnival would pass through, a maze of rides and games taking over a shopping mall parking lot for several days. I always found this remarkable. But in rural Wisconsin, the county fair is its own phenomenon. Many counties have fairgrounds, often with buildings used once a year to house exhibitions that range from cakes, cookies, and other baked goods to arts and crafts, and so many farm animals, a parade of domesticated creatures that embody millennia of breeding and illustrate humanity's interdependence with other species—cows, pigs, goats, sheep, chickens, rabbits, all displayed to the public, reared to perfection or specification, the fittest judged and awarded ribbons, then auctioned to the highest bidder.

The Minnesota State Fair is like a rural county fair on steroids, with attendance sometimes exceeding two million people over a twelve-day period in late August. A given day can see hundreds of thousands of people pass through. It's almost always busy. The day we went, cars lined up for miles as drivers desperately hunted for parking. After we finally found a parking spot, we loaded Aidric and Michaela into a double stroller, donned hats and dutifully covered them in sunscreen, then joined the hordes of people wandering through beer gardens, animal barns, carnival rides, and food tents that serve almost everything imaginable, often on a stick.

As we walked, I thought of Franz Boas, who in 1893 assisted with creating a series of anthropology exhibits at the Chicago World's Fair. In its time, the World's Fair was a colossal public event, buildings and halls assembled to display modern society's finest accomplishments in agriculture, science, technology, and industry. The Chicago World's Fair lasted six months, covered nearly seven hundred acres, and was visited by roughly twenty-seven million people. That year it was also known as the World's Columbian Exhibition, a celebration of the four hundredth anniversary of Christopher Columbus's arrival in the New World, a triumph of colonial discovery, at least for some Europeans. Anthropology exhibits were created to display native peoples living in mock villages, enacting what for fairgoers were strange cultural rituals. Boas aspired to introduce anthropology to the public, to display a growing knowledge of cultural variation. But the public educational component mixed uneasily with the reality of the time: mostly White attendees, who fashioned themselves as an embodiment of civilization, gazing at Brown and Black bodies on display, as if penned in at a zoo, living dioramas of primitive society.

Boas would go on to distance himself from such initiatives, but the practice of displaying non-White and non-Western people as exotic curiosities at fairs continued into the twentieth century. The 1904 World's

Fair in Saint Louis featured an entire village of the Igorot, a people of the Philippines, a colonized country recently taken over by the imperial exploits of the United States following the Spanish-American War. That fair also featured Ota Benga, a Congolese man who was displayed in a cage, along with apes, as an example of earlier stages of human evolution. The display of Benga communicated a racist social hierarchy, Africans alongside animals, superior White Americans gawking as they strolled from one exhibit to another. Set up as illustrations of human evolution and progress, the displays reinforced for a White public their claim to innate superiority.

In the early twentieth century, the message of racial and civilizational progress expanded beyond the celebration of technological innovation and beyond the display of an objectified, dehumanized non-Western Other. The eugenics movement turned the focus inward, scrutinizing the unfit within the body politic. State and county fairs became an important space for enacting this growing preoccupation with deficiency or impairment propagating from within. The 1908 Louisiana State Fair is thought to have been the first to host a "Better Babies" contest, an exhibit in which parents displayed their babies, who were then judged based on numerous criteria of desirability. Like the livestock in the next building over, White babies were measured and poked, their features compared and judged as healthy or superior, their mental acuity or personality assessed with intelligence tests. Over the next two decades, such contests spread through fairs in the Midwest and elsewhere, partly in a public health effort to promote pediatric care.[59] But child wellness efforts quickly intersected with eugenics, and health became overshadowed by themes of heredity and controlled reproduction. Winning children would receive a ribbon or certificate and be displayed like other prize-winning animals.

As a poster from the 1929 Kansas Free Fair stated, "How long are we Americans to be so careful for the pedigree of our pigs and chickens and cattle, and then leave the ancestry of our children to chance, or to 'blind' sentiment?"[60] That 1929 fair also featured a "Fitter Families" contest, the eugenic rationale extending from the reproduction of certain types of persons to the creation of ideal family types. The popularity of these contests and their routine appearance at state and county fairs in the early twentieth century illustrates the widespread acceptance of the beliefs central to eugenics, which were woven into popular culture and the recreational activities of the time. The exhibits and contests reinforced the idea that undesirable bodies and minds, the unfit and feebleminded, the racially problematic, could be easily identified and weeded out, and that those with superior features could and should be encouraged to reproduce for the benefit of society, linking family and national fitness.

Boas helped establish a new brand of anthropology that would famously challenge eugenics. But in other ways his work also tacitly perpetuated the racist and colonial power structures that shaped society and birthed the discipline of anthropology, the traces of which my profession continues to bear. Even as he challenged the assumption that certain immigrant groups were mentally defective, that indigenous peoples had innately "primitive" and feeble minds, that racial Others would dilute civilization, he celebrated their ability to "amalgamate" or assimilate into dominant White society, leaving Whiteness and colonialism largely unexamined.[61]

Similarly, in Boasian anthropology, cognitive disability or neurodiversity became nonissues. Mental deficiency, assumed by eugenicists to be race-based and transmitted in families across generations, was being blamed for all sorts of problems in Boas's time—poverty, crime, alcoholism, sexual promiscuity. In challenging the flawed science behind eugenics, Boas and his followers, such as Benedict, Mead, and Sapir, challenged the view that some groups were inherently impaired, that they would propagate disability across society, that they were fundamentally Other. But they sidestepped the issue of disability itself, the people being classified as feebleminded, the question of what such diversity means for understanding the human condition. They argued that mental deficiency is not innate among groups, then left its study to others.

Mead's groundbreaking *Coming of Age in Samoa*, for instance, includes a brief two-page appendix titled "The Mentally Defective and Mentally Diseased," in which she documents having observed imbeciles, idiots, and low-grade morons. "Without any training in the diagnosis of the mentally diseased and without any apparatus for exact diagnosis of the mentally defective," writes Mead, "I can simply record a number of amateur observations which may be of interest to the specialist interested in the possibilities of studying the pathology of primitive peoples."[62] Disability is present in her study of Samoan culture but relegated to an appendix—an afterthought.[63]

As Tiffani and I pushed our stroller and wandered through the Minnesota State Fair, only animals were on display. The anthropology exhibits of Boas and the once immensely popular Better Babies and Fitter Families contests were now faded memories. We walked past dozens and dozens of cows, close enough to touch them, to hear them breathe. The earthy aroma of their manure lingered far beyond their enclosures. We remarked on more varieties of bunny rabbits and poultry than I ever imagined existed. As we walked between sections of the fair, we were shoulder to shoulder with people.

Amid all of this, I found myself thinking largely of the varieties of humans around me. Were we the only ones, I thought? I was still working through the emotional impact of the diagnosis, a shock wave that scrambled my understanding not only of Michaela, but of the world we inhabit. Well-meaning doctors and friends had cued grief as the suitable feeling, but this didn't seem to fit. I thought of a colleague who had recently lost a twin infant during childbirth, and my feelings came nowhere close to the catastrophic anguish he experienced. My loss was that of an imagined future, not a child. I was coping not with loss, but with difference.

A sea of thousands of people coursed through the fairgrounds, and I was looking desperately for another child with Down syndrome.

That day I found none, except my own.

3 Institutions

When I was a child in the 1980s, my great-grandparents used to take me and my brother to see our Grandma Joan. My dad almost never came along. During the summer, it was a frequent, sometimes weekly outing that would take up most of the day. The forty-five-minute drive to Kankakee, south of Chicago, seemed to last forever, and felt even longer on the way back as rush hour set in. A black plastic compass, partially melted from car heat, was glued to the car dashboard, and saltine crackers were always in the glove box.

After a breakfast of Lucky Charms cereal and an episode of *Bozo the Clown* or *Transformers* cartoons, my Great-Grandma Rossi would load me and my brother and my great-grandfather into their car, folding and hoisting his wheelchair into the trunk. All my memories of my Great-Grandpa Rossi include him using a wheelchair. He had spent most of his prime laboring years helping to make ball bearings at an International Harvester factory on the South Side of Chicago, a steady, unionized job with good pay and benefits. But he also lost most of his ability to hear. In late midlife, he became ill and a lengthy stay in the hospital left him unable to walk on his own. When I was a boy, he could still move himself from his wheelchair to a sofa, where he would sit and watch baseball.

One day when I was about six years old, we arrived in Kankakee to find my Grandma Joan waiting just inside the front doors of her nursing home. She quickly walked to the car and my great-grandmother handed her two cartons of Marlboro cigarettes through the window, ten packs to a carton. She removed a single pack and hastily tore off the crisp cellophane wrapper, lifting open the paper lid to free a single cigarette, raising it to her lips. A lighter flashed in front of her face as she tugged on the spark wheel with her thumb, hardened steel grinding against flint, gas igniting in a small flame. Then she paced near the entrance to the nursing home, sitting on a bench and then standing, sitting again, standing, long drags followed by relieved exhales, smoke rising above her head. When she was done, she pressed the burning cigarette into an ashtray and walked over to greet me and my brother, watching from the back seats of the car, my great-grandparents still waiting in the front.

She opened the car door and gestured for me to step out. She knelt and embraced me, pulling me snugly against her warm body, burying her face in my neck. We remained like that. She held me tightly, gripping me. I couldn't get away. She rocked back and forth. "Oh, Tommy, Oh, Tommy, Oh, Tommy," she repeated, tobacco odor lingering in her straight, raven-black hair.

We took Grandma Joan to lunch at the usual place, a restaurant called The Little Corporal. It had red walls and blue upholstered booth seating, though we sat at a table to accommodate my great-grandfather's wheelchair. Pie and other desserts turned slowly in a bright, refrigerated display case. A large painting of Napoleon showed him in tight pants with what appeared to my childhood eyes an exceptionally large bulge. I ordered a breaded fish sandwich. Grandma Joan ended up outside most of the time, smoking. After lunch we went to a park next to the Kankakee River. It featured long, swooping swings and a dangerously tall spiral slide. My great-grandparents tossed old bread to ducks.

During the long drive home, we got stuck in traffic somewhere on the far South Side of Chicago. It was late in the afternoon. We inched forward, accelerating, slowing down, starting and stopping in a line of cars. As the car idled, we came up next to a black sports car driven by a gorgeous young woman. She lifted a cigarette to her mouth and took a long drag, blowing smoke out of the window.

The noise startled me. "Goddamn it, Peggy!" screamed my Great-Grandpa Rossi, referring to my great-grandmother by her nickname. He slammed his fists against the dashboard, the thud reverberating through the car, rattling the melted compass. "What the fuck!"

I was frightened. I had never seen my great-grandfather explode like this before, even when he hollered at the TV during baseball games. I had never heard him swear. "Goddamn it, Peggy! She is ruining her fucking life! She's so young! She's beautiful! I can't believe she is ruining her life! Smoking goddamn cigarettes!"

His tone was thick with remorse. He howled at the window as the pace of the cars increased, lamenting the demise of a young woman, the flow of traffic pulling her away, and there was nothing he could do.

.   .   .

My uncomfortable memories of Grandma Joan have imprinted in me a lasting curiosity about institutions. After my dad was born in 1955, his parents, Joan and Ronald Pearson, moved to a new home in suburban Alsip. They purchased the house through the GI Bill's home loan program, following my Grandpa Ron's service in the postwar occupation of Germany. He became a Chicago firefighter the year my dad was born. It was a 1950s success story, a young couple with a child in a new single-family home, benefiting from government programs and stable, unionized work. My Grandpa Ron continued to claim his parent's home address in the adjacent Chicago neighborhood of Mount Greenwood, the city residency allowing him to work as a Chicago firefighter, alongside his own father. Mount Greenwood is a largely White middle-class neighborhood known for racial segregation. In the 2016 election, it was the only neighborhood in Chicago where most voters supported Trump.

Shortly after my dad was born, his mom's behavior became increasingly erratic and violent. She pressed burning cigarettes against the bottoms of his feet and attacked her husband with a knife. As her mental health deteriorated, my dad was removed from her care and she was institutionalized at Manteno State Hospital, once the largest psychiatric hospital in Illinois and among the largest in the United States, located in rural Kankakee County, about thirty miles from the South Side of Chicago. Her husband soon left her, and my great-grandparents moved into the house in Alsip to raise my father. Grandma Joan was in and out of Manteno State Hospital until it was shuttered in 1985, sometimes living at home with her parents, sometimes living in halfway houses. She became a ward of the state and eventually lived permanently in a nursing home. My father lost his mother to mental illness. My great-grandparents lost their daughter. When Grandpa Rossi exploded at the driver smoking in the car next to us, he was likely mourning an emotional trauma he was otherwise unable to express.

Before my brother and I started kindergarten, my own parents moved into that Alsip house and took out a mortgage to build an attached apartment for my aging great-grandparents, who helped watch over me and my brother. My parents had married young, barely out of high school. When my brother Jim was born, my dad was twenty-one years old, my mom just nineteen. My dad took jobs for the city driving snowplows and hauling trash, then worked at a car dealership before using a family connection to get a job as an account manager at a trucking company. With two young children in tow, my mom finished her college degree and then worked as a special education teacher. My parents provided periodic assistance to my great-grandparents as Great-Grandpa Rossi's health declined, and my great-grandmother provided childcare, watching me and my brother so that my parents could work or go to class.

In my childhood memory, the Alsip house is gigantic, but really it was a small, midcentury bungalow. Thorn-covered rose bushes grew along the driveway and the fenced-in yard brought endless adventure for me and my brother. Overgrown pine trees crowded the front yard, and a wheelchair access ramp covered the house's front steps. By the time I was in second grade, my parents were able to sell the Alsip house to invest in an even bigger home in the distant suburbs, joining the phenomenon of suburbanization—prejudice-fueled White flight and a cycle of middle-class upward mobility enabled in part by real estate transactions. The wealth generated through access to GI Bill benefits and my great-grandfather's union pension has indirectly underwritten multiple generations in my family, and eventually my parents gifted me the down payment for my first home a couple years after I started working at UW-Stout in Menomonie.

As a child, I was told Grandma Joan had "gotten sick" shortly after my dad was born, then later that she had suffered a "nervous breakdown." She likely had postpartum depression and was eventually diagnosed with schizophrenia and bipolar disorder. She benefited greatly from antipsychotic drugs as they became more refined, but never returned home on a permanent basis. When my brother and I visited along with my great-grandparents, Grandma Joan was living in a long-term nursing home facility, where she remained the rest of her life. After my great-grandparents became frail with old age and then died, we rarely visited Grandma Joan. At some point, the state moved her to another facility in southern Illinois and my dad drove down to retrieve her ashes after she died in the early 2000s.

If Michaela had been born in Menomonie in 1944, the same year as Neil Erikson, it's likely she would have ended up at an institution that was then called the Northern Wisconsin Colony and Training School, located about thirty miles away in Chippewa Falls. Menomonie and Chippewa Falls, along with the larger city of Eau Claire, are connected historically and economically. They sit along intersecting rivers that once served the flourishing logging industry and comprise what is known locally as the Chippewa Valley. The Northern Wisconsin Colony and Training School originally opened in 1897 as the Home for the Feeble-Minded, the first of two state institutions to care for "feeble-minded and epileptic" children. Such places were envisioned as "custodial and training schools" where feebleminded children could learn basic skills. Eventually, perhaps, residents would be reintegrated into society, and at least they would be trained to be economically productive while under state care. Like other nineteenth-century asylums and similar institutions in rural areas, the Home for the Feeble-Minded was a working farm. Inmates produced food and other resources, making it partially self-sufficient. Labor was viewed as therapeutic.

In that period, Chippewa Falls, like nearby Eau Claire and Menomonie, was a small city trying to promote economic activities beyond logging and agriculture. Local officials aggressively lobbied for the state to develop the Home for the Feeble-Minded, offering several hundred acres of land at Silver Spring Park. About a mile and half outside the city limits, the location was close to town yet still remote, adjacent to the Chippewa River and surrounded by wooded hills and hundreds of acres of farmable land. Proximity to nature was viewed as healthful and rejuvenating. A rail line passing through allowed for a train station at the site, an artery to the outside world.

The plans in 1896 called for twenty buildings, including dormitories, boys and girls schools, barns, a hospital, a gymnasium, and the railway station, scattered throughout a "beautiful park."[1] British-born architect John Charles, based out of Menomonie, was originally hired to design the campus, which was anchored around an ornate administration building.[2] Photographs of the building, especially in its early years, show a large, pressed-brick structure with a wide stairway that leads up to an open front porch at the main entrance, which is flanked by two octagonal towers. The building design reflected the beautiful Georgian-revival architectural style of late nineteenth-century state institutions. Dormitories and other buildings, while consistent stylistically, were much more utilitarian in design.

John Charles had a reputation for designing asylums and other institutional buildings and left the imprint of his career throughout the region. In 1891, he designed the Dunn County Asylum for the Chronic Insane, what was then one of the most comprehensive asylums in the state, boasting capacity for 117 patients. It was located outside Menomonie, which in the nineteenth century was also the home of the Knapp, Stout and Company lumber empire, a world-renowned logging company. The lumber industry dictated much of the economic and political direction of Menomonie at that time and lumber baron James Huff Stout sat on the county board committee that founded the asylum.

Around the same time, the early 1890s, Stout used his immense wealth to establish the Stout Manual Training School in downtown Menomonie, right at the intersection of Broadway and Main Street. His school anchored the center of town, and the asylum was at the margins, parallel institutions that embodied emerging conceptions of normality. When the original wooden structures housing the Stout Manual Training School burned down just a few years after its opening, Stout contracted Charles to design a new school building. What is now called Bowman Hall was completed in 1898, a brick building featuring a 135-foot-high clock and bell tower and a 12-foot weathervane shaped like a quill feather. It's a homage to knowledge and innovation, and the bell, which chimes every fifteen minutes, can be heard miles away, an audible symbol of industrial efficiency and capitalist routine. The presence of the building is unmistakable.

The Home for the Feeble-Minded, the Dunn County Asylum, and Bowman Hall all have similar architectural styles, featuring dark-red brick exteriors with cut stone foundations, numerous arched windows, and prominent towers. But only Bowman Hall still stands today, as the hallmark of what is now the University of Wisconsin-Stout campus. Photographs of the clocktower dominate the university's present-day marketing and for many years the quill was part of its logo. My office is next door to Bowman Hall, and I pass the building daily. It is a celebrated historical landmark and millions of dollars have been spent on its restoration and maintenance. But few acknowledge its relationship to other structures and histories, the buildings created to confine the impaired and disabled, which were erased by time and neglect.

The Dunn County Asylum for the Chronic Insane was demolished in the 1970s, replaced by a modern county health center that now serves as offices for Dunn County Human Services. Menomonie itself has grown, with commercial and housing development expanding away from the historic downtown, reaching what was once the remote site of the asylum. In fact, it happens to be a short walk from my current house. When I stroll down the block with Michaela, we can gaze across a farm field, especially during the winter or in the spring before the corn is tall, and see some of the old buildings still on the site. One of my favored jogging routes takes me past the old asylum grounds and along the county farm once worked by asylum inmates. A few old outbuildings still stand—a power plant, a blacksmith shop, a large shed, a garage—some with broken windows and peeling paint, cluttered with debris. The shed and garage are still used by the county highway department to store tools and equipment. A potter's field is nearby, unmarked graves holding the remains of unclaimed asylum residents.

Though it is still operating, the Home for the Feeble-Minded is similarly a mere shadow of what it once was, a blend of old buildings and artifacts that hint at a troubled past. It was renamed the Northern Wisconsin Colony and Training School in 1922, its population peaking at over two thousand in the early 1960s as an overcrowded and underfunded state institution.[3] In 1976, it underwent another name change, reflecting the wave of transformations occurring as such institutions were down-sized and caretaking shifted to community settings and group homes, becoming the Northern Wisconsin Center for the Developmentally Disabled. In 1977, the population dropped below one thousand for the first time in nearly seventy years. It dropped below five hundred residents by 1990. By the early 2000s, the remaining 150 long-term residents were resettled into group homes or "community-based facilities."[4]

Today the Northern Wisconsin Center operates as a short-term treat-ment and assessment facility, overseen by the Wisconsin Department of Health Services. The larger campus hosts an awkward blend of public services, including Head Start, the Chippewa Valley High School, and the Veteran Housing and Recovery Program. An infirmary built in 1966 has been converted to a minimum-security state prison. Abandoned buildings and cottages sit empty and boarded up, surrounded by chain-link fences, put up decades ago to deter residents from wandering into the street. The original administration building designed by Charles appears to have been recently demolished, but several other historic buildings still stand.

On the east side of the campus, a path through an open grassy area leads under an arched footbridge built of stone and crumbling cement, once part of the system of walkways that allowed residents to enjoy the natural surroundings. The path sinks into a wooded area with gravel and dirt trails. Immense red and white pines mix with oak, maple, birch, and other trees and surround a clearing with wetlands and a narrow, twisting stream. The stream flows under the trail through a large drainpipe, each end of which is covered clumsily by latticed metal bed springs, the small ones found in a crib or child's bed. I suppose someone placed them there, repurposed from years past, to keep animals or perhaps people from crawling into the pipe. At the other end of the clearing the trail passes by piles of debris from demolished buildings, old dormitories where children once slept, possibly the remains of the administration building. A bit fur-ther is a cemetery, hidden away, lines of gravestones placed flat on the ground near a railroad track. Only names are inscribed on the plaques. No birth dates. No death dates. Just names, hundreds of names.

·   ·   ·   ·   ·

Alfred A. Wilmarth served as the first superintendent of the Home for the Feeble-Minded, appointed in January 1897, just months after he published his article "Heredity as Social Burden" in the *Journal of the American Medical Association.*[5] He was forty-two years old and a medical doctor in the prime of his career, having held positions as assistant superintendent of the Pennsylvania Home for the Feeble-Minded and assistant physician at the Pennsylvania State Hospital for the Insane. Like others during his time, he saw the deficiencies of the feebleminded as distinctly hereditary. While he dismissed John Langston Down's speculation about the racial degeneracy of "mongoloids," he suggested in 1899 that the "hereditarian 'taint'" of the condition, "caused by arrested brain development, or brain damage, could be passed down to later generations."[6] In addition to brain damage, Wilmarth speculated about the association of mental deficiencies with perceived moral failings, such as alcoholism or promiscuity, and saw heritability as playing a key role in reproducing these flawed traits.

Segregation could prevent the feebleminded from reproducing. The Wisconsin Home for the Feeble-Minded, in his vision, would be a "refuge" or island with "villages of the simple."[7] He maintained that the mentally deficient placed a burden on families and communities, and were better off under the care and charity of the state, where they could live cheerfully and develop to their fullest potential. The state would protect their right to be educated, "as far as practicable," he wrote, "to a wider field of usefulness, which is the only true road to a higher degree of happiness."[8]

Wilmarth felt a moral responsibility to care for feebleminded children. But this duty of care would also benefit society by removing them from it. By 1906, in reports to the State Board of Control, Wilmarth pleaded for additional resources in starkly eugenic terms, tapping into public anxieties about the uninhibited nature of the mentally defective. "The high grade imbecile is prolific," he wrote, echoing themes that would later reach a broad audience in books such as Goddard's *The Kallikak Family.* "This class do not remain unmarried. One woman frankly explained her third marriage by saying that she 'had no other way of getting a living'; a statement most pathetic, as such marriages forecast little happiness and children are born weak and are trained by incapable parents into incapable men and women." The feebleminded woman was perceived as hypersexualized, unable to resist her "animal passions," as one observer of the Wisconsin Home wrote, and thus a threat to herself and society.[9]

Wilmarth suggested that the uncontrolled reproduction of the mentally defective would be far more costly to the state than the cost of lifelong institutionalization. "The state can do no better service to this rising generation than to give this class the care it needs from its hands, to cut off this increase, so far as is possible. No woman should be allowed to become a mother of nineteen defectives, as is recorded in one case, or of half that number, which occurs in very numerous instances. The State must protect such women from themselves, and incidentally the public purse and public morality."[10] He promoted institutions as an essential tool to segregate the mentally defective from society in order to prevent them from reproducing. Beyond the institution, he advocated prohibiting marriage among the feebleminded. As state capacity to house people was pushed to the limit, he then called for sterilization as a more efficient strategy and became one of the procedure's most outspoken advocates.

Wilmarth's writing expressed anxiety about the transmission of "degeneracy," and he favored eugenic policies that would prevent those deemed undesirable from passing on their flawed conditions. Far from being fringe beliefs, in the early twentieth century such ideas had broad support among government officials and industry leaders and were propagated by scientists, medical doctors, and others who hoped to improve national wellbeing through selective breeding. Dozens of states contemplated or passed laws restricting marriage selection or adopted laws allowing for forced sterilization, particularly of "mental defectives."[11] In many cases, inmates on track to be released from asylums or other institutions were first required to undergo sterilization. In 1927, the U.S. Supreme Court in *Buck v. Bell* upheld the forced sterilization of Carrie Buck, an inmate of the Virginia State Colony for Epileptics and Feebleminded. She had been committed to the Virginia Colony after becoming pregnant at seventeen, the outcome of being raped by the nephew of her foster parents, for whom she did housework.[12] After the Supreme Court upheld the forced sterilization of "imbeciles" as constitutional, over thirty states ended up passing sterilization laws of some form. Over sixty-two thousand people were forcibly sterilized between 1927 and the 1960s.

Eugenics policies in the United States were praised by Adolf Hitler in his 1925 manifesto *Mein Kampf* and the Nazi regime adopted sterilization laws in 1933 "nearly identical" to those in the United States.[13] The Nazi policy of racial purification took eugenics beyond the management of reproduction and down the horrific path of "exterminating" groups perceived as a detriment to the nation. The Aktion T-4 "euthanasia" program, one of the first extermination programs adopted in Nazi Germany, targeted children diagnosed with perceived hereditary diseases such as "idiocy" and "mongolism," as well as other disabilities. Before the start of WWII, at least 5,000 disabled children were killed under the T-4 program. When war broke out, the program was expanded to adults. Between 70,000 and 95,000 disabled people were murdered before the program was officially stopped in 1941. People with "mental deficiencies" continued to be killed through the end of the war, likely doubling the number of T-4 victims.[14]

·   ·   ·   ·   ·

Wisconsin adopted its own sterilization law in 1913, focused on mental defectives. The procedure began at the Wisconsin Home two years later and continued into the 1960s. Roughly eighteen hundred people were sterilized in Wisconsin over five decades, with nearly five hundred officially recorded at the Wisconsin Home.[15] The law required "consent" of the patient, but potential "parole" or release from institutionalization became contingent on sterilization, and in cases where patients lacked the cognitive capacity to provide consent, family would be consulted. If family could not be reached, consent was presumed.

About 80 percent of people sterilized were women and the procedure acted as a mechanism of control in a society of unequal gender relations. Terms like "mentally defective" or "feebleminded" were broadly applied to women accused of transgressing social norms. Public calls to protect "motherhood" were common, and women were sometimes viewed as needing protection from themselves. Women across race and class lines were blamed for perceived social ills and targeted by extraordinary state interventions, though sterilization disproportionately impacted recent immigrants, poor Whites, Indigenous peoples, Black people, and people with disabilities.[16] Given that people with cognitive disabilities were and remain especially vulnerable to physical and sexual abuse, one can only wonder to what extent these women were, like Carrie Buck, victims of rape blamed for being "promiscuous" or "prolific."

As in Buck's case, children deemed "delinquent" and women perceived as transgressive were sometimes institutionalized under questionable circumstances. In 1923, Anna Lenz was admitted to the Wisconsin Home for the Feeble-Minded as an unmarried, twenty-nine-year-old woman after being blamed for another woman's mysterious death, accused of sending her poisoned chocolate through the mail. Lenz was thought to have epilepsy and worked in the region as a "hired girl" on local farms, her speech colored by a "nearly unintelligible German accent," a language heavily stigmatized following the First World War.[17] Authorities extracted a dubious confession from Lenz after several hours of interviewing. During the murder trial, they declared Lenz feebleminded and mentally unfit to stand trial, and she was institutionalized.[18] She lived at the Wisconsin Home for the Feeble-Minded for nearly seven decades until her death in 1990, even as employees there eventually acknowledged that she was not cognitively disabled.[19]

Wilmarth rationalized the state-sanctioned violence of sterilization in eugenic terms, disguised as science. "The certainty of heredity has been so thoroughly established," Wilmarth wrote in 1916, "that the tendency to transmit mental weakness, or instability, is no more to be disputed than the accuracy of the multiplication table."[20] In fact, anthropologists such as Boas routinely disputed this very assumption, and Mead, Benedict, and Sapir challenged it as well. Wilmarth's views, however, were considered by many government officials as scientifically sound and progressive, part of a strong welfare state system that would protect public health and engineer societal improvement.[21] Prominent intellectuals supported eugenics in Wisconsin. In 1914, Charles Van Hise, president of the University of Wisconsin, offered eugenics as one part of the scientific management of society to improve wellbeing: "We know enough about agriculture so that the agricultural production of the country could be doubled if the knowledge were applied; we know enough about disease so that if the knowledge were utilized, infectious and contagious diseases would be substantially destroyed in the United States within a score of years; we know enough about eugenics so that if the knowledge were applied, the defective classes would disappear within a generation."[22] Van Hise is often credited with coining the "Wisconsin Idea," a principle that emphasizes the contributions of public universities, especially scientific expertise, to government policymaking and the improvement of communities across the state. The Wisconsin Idea is still routinely invoked in broad terms to promote and defend public higher education in Wisconsin, though Van Hise's association with eugenics is largely ignored or forgotten.

Like the remnants of the county asylum and potters' fields near my home, the ghosts of this period are present if you look for them. In the early twentieth century, my own university, then called the Stout Institute, published syllabi and other materials to prepare teachers in elementary and high schools around the country, including materials on how to teach eugenics.[23] The university archivist discovered a 1913 syllabus on eugenics after I inquired about the history of disability on campus. The document is described as "an outline, suggested topics for discussion, and bibliography for reference and class work in Home and Social Economics." It's incredibly detailed and begins with topics such as "the law of natural selection" and "heredity" as factors in "social progress." Under a section on "problems related to the study of heredity," the syllabus includes "transmissible diseases," "racial poisons," "social conditions reacting disastrously upon the germ cells," "diseases and physical traits having a tendency to run in certain family strains," and "mental and moral traits appearing in certain family strains." A concluding section on "practical eugenics" lists methods of "negative eugenics," including "sterilization," "segregation," "restrictions on marriage of the unfit," and "state intervention for the protection of motherhood."

I was initially stunned to discover the document, but in retrospect I should not have been surprised. The history of my university reflects a historical reality that few people like to acknowledge. In the early twentieth century, higher education and academic research played an essential role in setting the boundaries of normalcy, defining stigmatized groups according to supposedly innate deficiencies that threatened social progress and national wellbeing. Universities expressed generic ideals of knowledge and understanding, but also elite, capitalist ideologies of innovation, improvement, and exclusion, advancing and disseminating practical fields of study, including eugenics.

Campus architecture also illustrates this ideology of "higher" education, with ornate buildings perched on hills, often with grand staircases making them physically accessible only to the able-bodied.[24] As buildings such as UW-Stout's Bowman Hall were erected in the centers of towns—the heart of community and economic life—what took shape on the margins was "the inverse or opposite of higher education," the asylums or schools for the feebleminded where people with disabilities, or those perceived as transgressive, were segregated and confined.[25] Ideological boundaries, the categories and types used to define human bodies and minds, were inscribed across physical and geographic space. These inverse institutions were frequently connected, directly and indirectly. Like James Huff Stout, economic and civic leaders often had a hand in founding both sets of institutions. Over the years, university students would visit and sometimes intern at asylums and at schools for the feebleminded. And, in the case of Menomonie, the architect John Charles designed the first buildings for my university, the old county asylum, and the Home for the Feeble-Minded, linking all three institutions.

Architectural design is never just a functional task.[26] Charles would have visited the proposed locations, imagined life there, and surely spoken with local officials and others involved in planning. He would have studied the roles of these institutions in social and economic development. Then he would have sat in his Menomonie office overlooking the lumber operations and mill pond, the same lake I look out at today from my office window, envisioning who would occupy the respective buildings, carefully drawing out his plans. He had to conjure in his imagination the types of people who would utilize the built environments and how physical spaces should be organized to facilitate certain behaviors, to foster certain minds, and to contain and discipline others.

Years later, the superintendents of those structures, of the bodies in them, turned to additional technologies of control, such as invasive surgeries like coerced sterilization. At the Home for the Feeble-Minded, amid a charming setting with apple orchards, pumpkin patches, and farm fields lined with corn and oats, surrounded by hills with tall pine trees swaying in the wind, the Chippewa River flowing steadily, superintendent Wilmarth sterilized young women, the procedure performed by local consulting surgeons.[27] Among the many photographs of the Home for the Feeble-Minded is one of a hospital operating table.[28] No people are shown in the photograph. I look at it and imagine that Wilmarth instructed his assistants to place sedated bodies upon the table. A surgeon sits down on a metallic stool and nudges himself closer, the stool legs scraping loudly against the black-and-white tile floor. He reaches up and pulls the bright lamp down. Quiet now. A still, almost lifeless body lays before him. A young woman. A child, really. Her chest rises slowly with each soft breath. The nurse stands to the side. Scalpel. You can hear the blade moving against pale skin. He slices into the girl's belly, exposing her fallopian tubes. He reaches in and severs them. First one side. Then the other. Irreversible.[29] She'll awake later in great pain, confused as to what has happened.

I imagine my daughter on that table and feel nauseated. The residue of this history is toxic. Into the first half of the twentieth century, universities like the one I teach at generated the science and the ideological rationale to justify eugenic policies and shape public perceptions of disability. Eugenics cast a wide net, with immigrants, racialized Others, criminals, sexual misfits, the insane and feebleminded all viewed as suspect. Intellectual renegades such as Margaret Mead challenged attitudes about sexuality and the racism of eugenics. But beliefs about "Mongolian idiocy" were so pervasive, so built into the architecture of society, that when her friend Erik Erikson sought her advice, even she conformed to them.

If anything is heritable, it's the traumas of history. The suffering caused by past classifications or "types"—feebleminded, idiot, moron, imbecile, mongoloid, insane—echo in the present, in the diagnosis, in the extra chromosome. They reverberate through the memories of my grandmother who lived in these institutions, who was lost to them. This past haunts us. It haunts me.

In 1944, I doubt I would have acted any differently than Erik Erikson or Margaret Mead.

We were on an airplane heading to Walt Disney World in Orlando, Florida when my brother Jim had a panic attack, the type of episode in which the sufferer fears certain death, is convinced of it. I suddenly thought of my Grandma Joan. We hadn't visited her in years. I was a senior in high school. Jim had been taking classes at an art college in downtown Chicago, commuting daily from the suburbs. This was probably the last time my parents took us on a family vacation. When we were young, they often took us to Disney World. The fictional, carefully sculped world of theme parks and movies provided an entertaining form of escapism, a way for consumers, if they could afford it, to gain access to idealized family experiences, to create memories. My parents loved taking us there as young children. They desired to relive those memories. But when you're eighteen or nineteen years old and accompanying mom and dad, the magic just isn't there anymore.

As the plane took off from O'Hare Airport, my brother and I found ourselves sitting in the front row of our section, directly behind first class. We had flown dozens of times in our lives, and it had never been stressful. Everything started out fine. Shortly after takeoff, as the plane groaned upward to its cruising altitude, we blasted through significant air turbulence, the kind where you're grateful to have a seatbelt on. Feeling as if my body was being pulled upward, I first grabbed the armrests, then put one hand up toward the ceiling as if to hold myself in place. Startled flight attendants braced themselves as the captain urged everyone to remain seated. The roller coaster ride had begun.

Jim grabbed my leg, gripping my shorts tightly in his fist. The initial rumble of turbulence began to subside, but the plane still rattled and shook as it passed through shifting air masses. He was breathing fast and overwhelmed with terror. I tried talking to him. He started to sob uncontrollably.

"It's okay, Jim. It's okay," I muttered. "We're going to be fine."

I didn't know what to do.

"Breath, Jim, take deep breaths. It'll be okay."

I held his hand. He squeezed mine so hard it hurt. We held hands as he cried. My older brother, my protector from high school bullies, a stalwart source of support, wept uncontrollably. Eventually he calmed.

After this episode I noticed other signs of distress. Trivial fears or worries escalated and became the intense focus of relentless anxiety: weather, health, sharks. Not that we visited the ocean much, living as we did in Illinois, but the one time we did in college, he wouldn't go near the water. A year later, we both took classes at a community college. As we drove to campus one day he seemed to have another panic attack. He gripped the door of the car so hard I thought he would rip off the handle. When he finally let go, I noticed his hands shaking.

He was often anxious and had trouble focusing. He lost a significant amount of weight. I thought maybe he was on drugs. At community college we took an earth science course together. A grandfatherly instructor told stories about vacationing in the Smoky Mountains and screened lots of films. Exams assessed information from the textbook. It was the only class Jim passed that semester because I did his work for him. After weeks in which he barely slept and after he had failed most of his classes, mom took him to the doctor. He was diagnosed with Graves' disease and treated for hyperthyroidism. This explained most of the symptoms and he improved after that.

Life has a way of reconnecting you with the past when you least expect it. Roughly ten years later I went through a rough patch that exposed a realm of psychological forces I had barely acknowledged, but that now sit with me, in the background of my mind, a reminder of emotional vulnerability, of a family legacy perhaps—of how we all experience disabling conditions over the course of our lives, and depend on others for support.

There was no one specific trigger, just a slow turning point, a stroll along the precipice and back. After several years of graduate school in Binghamton, New York, and after six months of fieldwork in El Salvador, I was lucky to win a grant to continue my dissertation research for a year in Costa Rica. It was an amazing experience. The grant allowed me to rent a small house near the University of Costa Rica in San José and paid my living expenses for a year. I can't say my research was groundbreaking or even all that useful, even though my project felt interesting and relevant, and generated some publications in respected academic journals.[30] But on a personal level the fieldwork experience was incredibly enriching. For a brief time, I felt connected to a network of other young people in their twenties and thirties engaged in social activism and working in NGOs to support Costa Rica's environmental movement. I also linked up with a group of locals and expats who met every Friday for pickup soccer, an hour or two of intense competition followed by a night out at a bar. My social life revolved around a diverse array of young, educated activists in a cosmopolitan setting, and I traveled widely through a country of stunning natural beauty. Every week seemed like a new adventure.

Amid all this, I experienced a difficult breakup with my long-term girlfriend after years of contemplating a shared future. Fieldwork is known for being hard on relationships—time and distance separate people, as does the distance that accompanies the experience of becoming emotionally invested in a new and different set of friendships, of moving between different cultural worlds. In my case we tried to make it work and my girlfriend spent several weeks in Costa Rica. But she was at a crucial juncture of her own career development, finishing law school and attempting to pass the bar exam. It was simply impractical and unfair of me to think she would interrupt her life to join my fieldwork venture. It was months in the making, maybe longer, but eventually our relationship unraveled.

After my grant money ran out, my fieldwork was done and I had to finish writing my dissertation. If I could have afforded it, I would have stayed in Costa Rica. Instead, I returned to the United States. My prospects for funding in Binghamton had dried up and I was already sitting on tens of thousands of dollars of student loan debt that had accumulated over the years, so I ruled out more loans to fund dissertation writing. At thirty years old, I found myself moving back into my parent's house in the suburbs of Chicago. My younger brother was eleven years old at the time. I felt alone and isolated, living in a bleak setting of uniform single-family homes occupied by dull middle-aged White people and their spoiled elementary school children.

I didn't realize I was struggling. My mind would latch onto worries that seemed logical, that had a loose anchor in lived experience, but then became amplified beyond explanation. Initially the thoughts focused on health. Jim once made a passing comment about a mole on my shoulder, which had been there my entire life, but I convinced myself beyond a shadow of doubt that it must be skin cancer and I would certainly die. A doctor assured me it wasn't. Then I started having chest pains. When I was in Costa Rica, my uncle had died suddenly of a massive heart attack. Most of the men on my mom's side of the family have had heart issues, and I convinced myself I was next. A trip to the ER and a battery of tests provided temporary comfort (on two separate occasions, with two differ-ent doctors). But the anxiety redirected itself, a pulse of thoughts that were always there, moving through your head, a hum that became impos-sible to block out, jumping from one issue to the next. I started thinking about harming my younger brother. The thoughts would creep in, alarm me, and to cope I would ponder plunging a steak knife into my forearm, through the two bones directly above my wrist. This cycle of thoughts would play out endlessly.

One evening I stood in my parent's kitchen holding a knife. I pushed the tip against the skin on my inner wrist. I pressed a little harder and contemplated the pain. I imagined the warm blood, first a trickle, then a steady flow. The image provided a brief distraction from the anxiety. Then I called my brother and told him what I was doing.

"I know what you're thinking," he said. "I'm on my way."

I put the knife down and waited for him outside. When he arrived, I got in his car, and we just started driving and talking. He described what I was experiencing, the constant cycling of anxiety-invoking thoughts, the stream that becomes impossible to shut out, that plays in the background throughout the day. He acknowledged that he had experienced the same thing, since high school in fact. Your mind generates these awful scenar-ios, he explained, of harming yourself or others, not because you want to do that, but because it's such a horrible outcome. Sometimes your anxiety focuses on those you care about, those you love most.

The explanation made sense to me. We continued driving, continued talking, and ended up in our childhood neighborhood in Alsip, which we had not visited in decades. We found the house our dad grew up in, the one we had lived in with our great-grandparents. The wheelchair ramp was gone, as were the rose bushes. We reflected on the trips to see Grandma Joan in Kankakee. We retraced the route we used to walk to elementary school. We talked about the kids we used to play with. About family. About change.

"You see," said Jim as he dropped me back off at our parents' house. "You can do it."

"Do what?" I asked.

"What were you thinking about this whole time?"

I had been thinking only about the topics of our conversation. I had been distracted from my anxiety. It felt like relief, and his point was that the flow of uncontrolled worry did not have to dominate me.

After that experience, I sought out counselling. I talked very little about it with my parents or friends, fearful of the stigma and judgment. My doctor prescribed some anxiety medications, which I tried but didn't like, since they caused uncomfortable side effects. The counselor I saw recommended an approach called cognitive behavioral therapy—basically, learning to manage anxiety not by ignoring it, but by becoming aware of problematic thoughts and then redirecting, focusing on what you can control, and so on. In my experience, it was straightforward, but took years of practice. My ability to manage anxiety improved along with my life circumstances. Several months after moving back to my parent's home to write my dissertation, I got a part-time adjunct teaching job at Roosevelt University in downtown Chicago. I did it mostly for the experience and for the opportunity to plug into a familiar academic community. I loved having a campus to travel to and having access to the university resources, sitting long hours in the library that overlooked Lake Michigan, writing my dissertation. I soon met Tiffani, who was then a graduate student at DePaul University. Before long, I was spending most of my time downtown, often at her northside apartment in Lake View, in the historic Boys Town neighborhood. As I was teaching at Roosevelt, writing my dissertation, and dating Tiffani, I also lined up a tenure track job for the following academic year at UW-Stout. If anything helps you manage anxiety and cultivate better mental health, it's the sense of security fostered by a string of good things happening in your life.

As my life became more grounded and my post-fieldwork plans clear, Jim's became more unsettled. He continued to struggle with his own anxiety, which worsened after his children were born and the stressors of life intensified. A few years after I moved to Menomonie to work at UW-Stout, he called me out of the blue. He couldn't take it anymore. The constant worry about his own health. The constant fear of something awful happening. He wasn't sleeping. Couldn't focus. The flow of anxiety, the stream of thought, always there, echoing in your mind even as you contemplate or discuss other topics, the obsessive thoughts of self-harm, or harming those you love most. When he hung up the phone, I thought for sure he was going to kill himself. I called my dad, who headed out to find him.

Jim drove himself to the emergency room, to my immense relief. They admitted him to the psychiatric ward, where he spent three days. He recounts it as an eye-opening experience, an opportunity to observe other people struggling amid psychotic episodes, some with their lives ensnared in substance abuse or other self-destructive behaviors, the sorts of things that destroyed my Grandma Joan. He came to see his own circumstances as vastly preferable and realized he wasn't suicidal but struggling with severe anxiety. It gave him a chance to step out from his day-to-day life, akin to the fieldwork experience, and to see it from a different perspective. Hospitalization also connected him with well-trained doctors and psychiatrists who supported him over subsequent years with the assistance of medications and therapy. If it had been the 1950s, he might have been institutionalized, like our grandmother, with an uncertain future. Instead, he was provided with mental health resources and supports, tools to move forward with his life. He received a formal diagnosis of obsessive-compulsive disorder, with an emphasis on the obsessive side of that condition, a form of anxiety disorder in which the mind fixates on irrational worries and thoughts, playing them repeatedly, unrelentingly, until it's overwhelming. The goal, as he had intuitively advised me years before, is not to ignore it, but to identify it, to call it out, to nurture it, to reveal its irrational character.

It never leaves entirely but fades into background noise.

.   .   .   .   .

We all experience tough times and vulnerability. It could be sickness or injury. It could be mental health. But impairment is part of life. We can ignore it, render it invisible, shroud it in silence and stigma, or we can acknowledge our common humanity and support each other. The path to such acknowledgment and mutual support is not simple, however.

As I absorbed the reality of Michaela's diagnosis in those initial months, my perception became subject to a history of classifications, and my daughter became the subject of classification. Like history, language has a powerful grip on consciousness. We became ensnared in a new and unfamiliar discourse, a web of meanings that marked Michaela as different, in contrast to other people deemed normal.

Medical diagnosis is more than a description of reality. Diagnoses are categories filled with meaning, and the definitions of these categories reflect historical circumstances. Like our understanding of Down syndrome, psychological diagnoses have evolved considerably, often in relation to changing ideas about human differences. As anthropologist Roy Grinker writes in his book *Nobody's Normal,* "judgments about mental illnesses have come from our definitions of what, at different times and places, people consider the ideal society and the ideal person."[31] Vulnerability is real, but how people make sense of this, and how it's judged, is the subject of cultural change.

During a visit to Chicago not long after Michaela was born, Jim and I were sitting with our parents around the kitchen table, talking and laughing. It was the end of the day, and Aidric and Michaela were already in bed. I was home. Conversation was random and jovial. My brother pulled out his phone and sifted through photographs of his own kids, thumb swiping across the phone's glossy surface, stopping on an image of one of his two sons, who in the photograph is standing and smiling, modeling a new set of eyeglasses. "He's my *special* kid," my brother said jokingly, emphasizing the word "special."

Another time, our children played joyfully in the living room. Aidric and his cousins had recently watched part of a gymnastics competition on television, inspiring them to unleash their own routines, bouncing and tumbling across the room, falling off furniture and banging into each other.

"Maybe they'll be in the Olympics one day," I commented.

"Yeah," responded Jim sarcastically, "the *Special* Olympics."

These were remarks about our "typical" kids, not intended as insults. It was suddenly clear to me, however, that disability serves as the foil to poke fun at their banal normalcy and to mark them as such. *They are not Olympians, but at least they are normal.* These sorts of comments do the heavy lifting of unconscious bias, defining the categories, placing kids inside or outside the imagined sphere of normality.

It's like the stigma and sense of shame around mental illness that leads people to ignore their suffering, to hide their struggles, in an effort to be perceived as normal.[32] Similar to ignoring my own mental health, I'm sure many times in my life I had engaged in such banter, calling people or ideas "retarded" or "idiotic," or referring to people or situations as "crazy" or "insane," not recognizing the ideological work being performed, a hidden history conjured into the present, cloaked as harmless teasing or benign remarks. Not long ago, such ideologies rationalized the violence of institutional confinement and forced sterilization.

Now here I was, an outsider for the first time, looking at my brother, a person with whom I have shared my most vulnerable moments, as I would an abrasive stranger, realizing my daughter needed protection in ways I had never imagined.

4 Potential

Michaela's birth enrolled us in a system. I suppose this is true of all infants. They are issued a birth certificate and their existence is fully acknowledged by the administrative state. Eventually they receive a social security number. They are officially accounted for.

A newborn also enters a less-bureaucratic social and cultural system, a family network and community that embraces, symbolically, at least, the new member. This social acknowledgement of personhood often begins prior to birth, with events such as baby showers or, in recent years, gender reveal parties. With our first child, we were the recipients of two different baby showers. Friends in Menomonie hosted the first, attended by colleagues and friends, most affiliated with the university. We ate food and eventually cake, other people's kids played on a swing set, and I sat with Tiffani as we opened gifts, an array of clothes, infant-care items, and books, lots and lots of books.

A couple weeks later my parents hosted a second baby shower for us at a golf course country club in the Chicago suburbs. Flat fairways curved gently around squatty trees, sand traps, and a retention pond, stocked with fish. Much of my parents' extended family attended, including many people I had not seen in years and whose names I often struggle to remember. We ate catered food and more cake, and again opened a pile of gifts, including some of the costlier items such as a crib and a wooden highchair from Eddie Bauer. On the table where guests placed their gifts, my mom displayed a framed photograph of me when I was a toddler. In the photo I'm wearing white overalls with red pinstripes and a solid red shirt underneath. I'm sitting alongside Jim, who has blue pants and a short-sleeved shirt with horizontal red and blue stripes. We are looking away from the camera but smiling. With a digital camera, I took a photo of the framed picture. In the days when we suspected Michaela might have Down syndrome, I studied it closely, comparing my features with hers, especially the ears. Michaela has small ears, tucked closely against her head. In the photo mine are much bigger, and stick out from underneath long, wavy brown hair.

The presence of the photo at the baby shower invoked linkages from one generation to the next, the pending birth of a baby representing not just biological reproduction but the reproduction of so much more—a family system. The baby shower was a ritual of class and kinship status, an exchange of gifts and wealth that reinforced a larger kin network and celebrated all the trappings of the modern nuclear family. For first-time parents such as me and Tiffani, it served as a rite of passage, facilitating our transition to parenthood. The identity and mindset of "parent" is something that unfolds gradually, and such events help it along. The gathering represented the symbolic birth of a family unit, with a larger community acknowledging the offspring-to-be. We also got lots of stuff.

With Michaela, our second, such events were more subdued. We had all the stuff already, and we had the identity, so there were no baby showers. Tiffani and I declined to find out the biological sex of any of our children before birth, so a gender reveal party was never even considered. On the day of her birth, my parents rushed up from Chicago to help with Aidric. They took him to the park and swam with him for hours at their hotel pool. Aidric sat on my dad's lap, reading stories. After a couple days, they left. As Tiffani and I settled into the possibility of Down syndrome, everything around us seemed to pause. When the diagnosis became official, there was a brief period in which the norms and rhythms of family life felt like they were in question. I wondered if my parents would feel disappointment. I feared the judgement of my extended family. I thought my life would become an endless cycle of medical appointments and therapy sessions. I truly had no idea what parenting Michaela would mean for us and assumed it would radically transform our family life. It didn't.

My parents and extended family, in their own ways, were supportive. Even if they felt uncertain or confused, Michaela's status as part of our family was never in question. Down syndrome does in fact increase the risk of some health issues, particularly heart problems, so our pediatrician ordered a series of evaluations with specialists, including an echocardiogram. Early on this created the expectation that we would embark on a path of frequent visits to medical doctors. I recall sitting with Michaela as a technician generated ultrasound images of her heart chambers, contemplating a life of appointments and procedures. But this has yet to occur. Her heart was fine.

Michaela, in fact, had no serious health issues as a baby. As recommended, in the early months we took her to an ear, nose, and throat specialist, to an audiologist, and to a pediatric ophthalmologist to screen for vision issues. Her eyesight was fine, but she did have a slight "wandering eye," one of her eyes appearing to drift out as she attempted to focus. It was barely noticeable to me. The solution was intermittent patching of the other eye, to strengthen the one that drifted. Her tear ducts also tended to clog, making her prone to eye infections, a potential consequence of having a slightly flattened facial profile. She had a procedure to have her tear ducts probed, resolving the issue.

Other than that, to date Michaela has been our healthiest, least accident-prone child. Aidric and Zora, by contrast, have both visited the ER multiple times for everything from a suspected seizure to respiratory distress, gaping head wounds, and a tongue laceration. Watching a doctor sew your kid's tongue back together is unforgettable. If I've learned anything as a parent so far, it's how to respond calmly to health emergencies and cope with the emotional toll of periodic hospital visits. Kids are resilient, but also dependent on others for their care and survival. The same goes for adults.

Despite all the manuals saying that Down syndrome makes a child more medically fragile, we've been lucky so far with Michaela. The only exceptional thing we had to do after Michaela was born was register her for our county-run "early intervention program," Birth-to-3, geared toward that period before children qualify for services such as speech or physical therapy through the school district. Our pediatrician had recommended it and we assumed it was just something that parents in our situation were supposed to do. We asked to sign up as soon as possible and were contacted in the days after Michaela was diagnosed. Therapists and a teacher started coming to our house when Michaela was barely a month old.

I recognize this can be useful for some children. Identifying and addressing developmental disabilities early can have lifelong implications. Some developmental disabilities become visible only gradually over the first months or years as children approach expected milestones, and quickly connecting with a community-based support system is crucial. But in our case, it was a bit silly. Michaela was too young and her development progressed too rapidly for her to really benefit from any of this just after birth. She readily nursed and in the first weeks could lift and turn her head and do just about anything else you would expect of a new baby.

It irritated me in those first several months when I had to clean the house and look presentable so that someone could come over and play with Michaela for an hour while I sat there and tried to engage in small talk. At that early stage, the therapists struggled to identify specific goals to work toward, because it was difficult to identify any significant "delays." And we never understood what the "teacher" did, though I gather she served as a case manager. Every time they asked what goals we wanted them to work on, we responded by saying, "Do whatever you need to do so that she can go to college someday."

In many ways, Michaela has been fortunate, and our need for home-based therapy wasn't extensive at the time. But I didn't realize that we were benefiting from a system of support and services that barely existed when I was born, and that was unimaginable in Neil Erikson's world.

. . . . .

It's unclear to me what motivated Margaret Mead to advise Erik Erikson to institutionalize Neil. Looking back, it seems so unethical, so narrow-minded, and so opposed to the type of cultural anthropology that Mead championed.

Throughout her career, she challenged Western assumptions about the universality of human behavior. She argued that culture, not biology, accounted for behavioral differences. This meant acknowledging and valuing the many ways of being human. Even gender and sexuality, so often assumed to be fixed or determined by underlying biology, are molded by culture, the biology of human reproduction or embodied variation shaped by social systems, given symbolic meaning that ultimately informs human experience. Biology is a blank slate on which culture takes shape.

"If we can find out how human beings differ, when they start out so much the same," said Mead, "we'll know a lot about the potentialities of human nature."[1]

This reflects the influence of Franz Boas, Mead's mentor. He had emphasized the underlying "psychic unity" of humanity, a basic assumption of his approach that has shaped anthropologists' study of culture ever since. Boas argued that despite perceived differences of race or nationality, people everywhere share underlying cognitive structures on which variations in language and culture are built. The resulting cultural relativist framework provided a powerful antidote to claims about the innate qualities of different peoples, but it also rendered neurodiversity invisible in the work of Boas and his followers.

Perhaps this was part of the problem, then. For all the power and openness of Mead's anthropological perspective, the cultural relativism that provided such an important challenge to the eugenics movement of the early twentieth century failed to account for disability, especially intellectual or cognitive disability. While many people become disabled over time, through accident or age, from a Boasian perspective they came into this world as part of that blank slate of psychic unity. Some people, however, are indeed *born* with cognitive disability. It is innate. Essential. Biologically determined. It is the very thing anthropologists in the Boasian tradition like to question at every turn. This has consequences for how anthropologists account for disability—or just ignore it—in their studies of cultural variation.

"If we maintain that all cultures are made by humans who have roughly the same mental capacities," explain present-day anthropologists Patrick

McKearney and Tyler Zoanni, "then people who appear to lack such abilities would seem to be, at best, at the margins of culture. Anyone seen to have a significant impairment of the cognitive equipment that enables the rest of us to engage in society becomes hard to study anthropologically."[2] And it becomes tempting to discount their humanity—to just ignore their place in humanity—since their existence complicates a very basic premise of modern anthropology.

The truth is, Michaela *does* differ from me, from others, in very fundamental, biological ways. I found myself confronting this idea a couple years after she was born, when I was lecturing about language and culture to my introductory cultural anthropology class. I was trying to explain the arbitrariness of language, in simple terms, and how language is much more than just a system of communication. *It's a system of symbols,* I said, through which we represent the world we experience, through which we color it with a tapestry of meaning. And the system or language one speaks is not innate—you are not born with it, rather, you learn it through socialization. *If you had been born in a different country,* I told my students, *you would have learned a different language, acquiring it in the first few years of life. All of us have the same capacity to learn language, the same underlying cognitive architecture to learn this complex system of representation, but a particular language—like culture—is something we obtain. The language itself is not innate.*

This is where I found myself stumbling, suddenly second-guessing myself. Michaela was not acquiring language like her brother had. She was using some utterances, but we had also begun learning American Sign Language to help things along, since it was clear that spoken language would be difficult for her. She was not mastering the basic grammatical structures and experiencing the flood of new vocabulary as other two- and three-year-old kiddos *just start doing.* Difficulty with verbal language is common among children with Down syndrome. Woven into every cell of Michaela's beautiful body is that extra twenty-first chromosome, a building block of life, her life, that imprints itself in characteristics she shares with others *like her,* not like me. Yes, she looks like me, but she also looks different. She thinks differently. Her relationship to language is different.[3] Underneath we're all the same, Boas had emphasized, his psychic unity knitting humanity into one fabric. We all have the same cognitive architecture to acquire language, I had told my students . . . except, except, I suddenly realized, some of us just don't.

Where does my daughter fit into this?

.   .   .   .   .

The reality, too, is that in 1944 when Neil Erikson was born, when Mead was called upon to consider his place in the world, institutionalization was routine, especially for children with Down syndrome. Children displaying the features of a so-called mongoloid were often identified at birth. Doctors frequently recommended immediate separation from the mother. They assumed institutionalization would be necessary at some point in the child's life and wanted to prevent strong bonds that would only make the inevitable all that more difficult. Many professionals at the time invoked a moral imperative to protect mothers from the perceived strain and hardship of raising a disabled child at home. It would be unfair to siblings, they suggested, and ruin the family. They commonly invoked what anthropologist Rayna Rapp calls the trope of alienated kinship, describing a "mongol infant" as lacking family resemblance with its parents, a pathological description that cast the newborn as alien or inherently different.[4] Tiffani and I encountered this same alienating urge when our pediatrician compared our features with Michaela's as her blood was drawn for genetic testing, speculating about her chromosomes, mumbling about a potential simian crease.

Mead, it seems, was sympathetic to concerns about the impact of a disabled child on family life, which seems ironic at first glance. Mead's own life was unorthodox and challenged the gender conventions of her era. She left her first husband as a young woman and traveled to Samoa. She met her second husband, an anthropologist, on the transoceanic voyage home after her fieldwork expedition. She met her third husband, also an anthropologist, while conducting fieldwork in New Guinea with her second husband. She was married and divorced three times over the course of her life. During decades when transgression of heterosexual norms was strongly policed in American society, Mead also cultivated intimate partnerships with women, most notably her mentor Ruth Benedict, who died in 1948, and her collaborator Rhoda Métraux, with whom Mead lived from 1955 until her death in 1978. Over the course of her life, Mead was a successful, professional woman, outspoken and independent, in an era when mainstream ideologies of family emphasized women's roles as doting mothers, deferential wives, and dutiful homemakers.

Despite living a life that seemed to challenge American norms around gender, sexuality, and family, her monthly columns for *Redbook* magazine, which she wrote with Métraux's assistance from 1962 until 1978, tended to reinforce mainstream views.[5] Mead was often understood to champion a more traditional notion of motherhood, anchored in the context of heteronormative marriage that saw women as natural homemakers. In the early 1960s, Mead discouraged her readers from engaging in premarital sex and described college education as a kind of "disaster insurance" for young women who might need to earn a living until they got married. Once married, they would obviously prefer to stay at home and raise children.[6] In one column, she responded to a reader question about "caring for and educating retarded children in primitive societies" by calling attention to the presumed toll on mothers, who would need "tremendous energy just to keep alive a seriously ailing or incapacitated child."[7] Mead's life may have been radical, but some of her advice to millions of young American women was not.

Mead's views about gender in American society evolved over the 1960s and 1970s and increasingly aligned with the feminist movement of that period, but her concern with the structure of family life amid the tumultuous social and economic changes of the modern era remained a constant theme. She often spoke about the isolation of the nuclear family, parents raising children without the support of a wider kinship network. "We take young people too young to be parents and tuck them into a strange suburb and make them responsible for everything," she said.[8] They are put into "a box" and an "impossible" situation.

In the non-Western societies she studied, family life was commonly embedded within extensive kin networks that structured the larger community. People's lives and identities were enmeshed in kinship systems, which could be constraining in some ways but also provided an important resource for addressing other challenges, such as childrearing. "It takes a village to raise a child," as the presumed African proverb goes.[9] And for millennia this is how human societies dealt with the work of social reproduction—as a collective, working together, sharing resources, ensuring group survival.

Americans, though, have a way of isolating one another. "We have burdened every small family," Mead wrote in 1977, "with tremendous responsibilities once shared within three generations and among a large number of people—the nurturing of small children, the emergence of adolescents into adulthood, the care of the sick and disabled, and the protection of the aged . . . obligations that traditionally have been shared within a larger family and wider community."[10] Mead was not anticipating the 1980s Reagan-era grumbling about the so-called demise of the traditional family. She was describing structural changes in modern industrial society that disproportionately impact women, especially in the work of caring for children or others and the labor of maintaining a household.

I've experienced this in my own family life. When I was a kid, my great-grandparents lived with us and routinely helped with childcare as my parents worked or went to school, especially when Jim and I were little. As they aged, the balance shifted, my parents providing more and more care for them. Mom and dad were sandwiched by the labor of simultaneously caring for children and for grandparents of advanced age. When my great-grandparents reached their eighties, their health needs became too complex and overwhelming. Grandpa Rossi spent the last few years of his life in a nursing home, frail and increasingly lost to dementia. I recall visiting him near the end, my first or second year of college, and finding him lying in his own feces, smeared on white bed linens. Grandma Rossi hung on at home slightly longer, but also spent her final years in a nursing home, overtaken by what seemed like paranoia and dementia before she died in a hospital intensive care unit. For all its strengths, Mead observed, in industrial society the nuclear family is poorly equipped to deal with the challenges of the human life cycle, and the support systems we've created to fill those gaps, such as nursing homes, can seem little more than a gateway to isolation and the relentless erosion of dignity until there is nothing left but a skeletal body covered in shit.

My parents are relatively young, and my grandparents have all passed, so for the time being I don't have to contemplate how to care for elders as well as my children. But my family—me, Tiffani, and the kids—face other challenges that Mead was drawing attention to when she said families are put into *impossible situations* without adequate support. We moved to Wisconsin for work, and are separated from parents, siblings, aunts and uncles, and cousins, some of them in Illinois and some in Utah. I'll admit, sometimes this is nice, especially when we dodge the dramas of obligatory family gatherings, the relentless pressures to accommodate expectation (to decide which set of relatives to visit on Christmas Eve or other holidays, for instance). But this also means we lack access to a ready-made kin network, a support system that others in my family can call on in a moment's notice. Nobody to watch our kids while we work or at random times, no one to go visit when we are just tired and could use an extra set of parental eyes, no one who feels that familial obligation to be a little more helpful with the slog of childcare. It's just me and Tiffani, with three kids, all the time, always outnumbered.

Since we both work full time, this means we've spent a small fortune in childcare for our small children. In 2019, the average cost of daycare in Wisconsin was $12,597 per year, more than undergraduate tuition at the state's flagship university.[11] Before our oldest started kindergarten, we spent one year with *three* children in daycare. Don't get me wrong, we are both lucky to have secure, decent-paying jobs at the university, with good health insurance, and I know childcare costs can be even higher in other parts of the country. But—and there's always a *but*—we are both employed at a lower-tier public higher education institution that has been systematically defunded in recent decades. Benefits have gradually eroded, and raises are hard to come by. The value of our salaries has been further reduced by the school loans we each took out decades ago to pay for our respective college degrees, which at the time seemed logical, since a college degree, we were told, is a middle-class ticket to the American Dream. But it has also meant a lifetime of debt. In our early forties, we are both still paying off student loans and have zero savings. When we started having children, we were weighed down by decades-old school debt while taking on the astronomical cost of daycare. My parents were sandwiched by the care-work of a multigenerational household; we were sandwiched by still paying for our own college educations while dishing out for the early childhood educations of our children. I know other families face more challenging scenarios than me and Tiffani—dealing with unemployment, health crises, or the many other inequities of our society—but our family life, unfolding as it is in Mead's metaphorical box, is still plain exhausting, the labor and financial strain of childcare a source of persistent tension between me and Tiffani.

When Mead advised Erik Erikson to send his infant son Neil to an institution in 1944, it's possible she reasoned that this would protect both Joan and her family, perhaps reduce the tensions of family life or keep things manageable. Joan was already the mother of three other children and the wife of a respected psychologist who was emerging as a significant intellectual figure—an expert, quite remarkably, on the psychological development of children. But Erik Erikson was enmeshed in a tradition of psychoanalysis that, like the Boasian commitment to a psychic unity of humankind, sought to understand how the environment in which a child is raised creates deviations from a presumed "normal" mind. A child born different fell outside of this framework. Lawrence Friedman, the biographer of Erik Erikson, recounts Mead's role as pivotal in Erikson's decision to "protect" his family from the "horrors" of a disabled child, as he puts it. "Mead had no doubts about the proper course for Neil," Friedman writes. "The hospital doctors were right, she told Erik." Raising Neil would "not benefit the children or family stability. Neil had to be institutionalized, Mead insisted, so that Joan would not form an attachment to him."[12]

Sociologist Allison Carey explains that during the 1940s, most medical professionals argued that "children with disabilities wreaked havoc on the family and placed a particular strain on the mother."[13] This narrative became dominant as eugenic rationales for institutionalizing children fell out of favor in the wake of World War II. Families, especially White, middle-class families, were increasingly understood to be smoothly functioning when women fulfilled their role as nurturing caregivers and when they identified with the professional accomplishments of their husbands. A disabled child threatened to undermine this equilibrium, demanding all the mother's time and energy, overwhelming her emotionally to the detriment of others under her care. The increased childcare responsibilities and emotional burdens would threaten to erode the husband's professional success as well. Yet even as this narrative of protecting the family replaced overt eugenic rationales, a scientifically accurate explanation for Down syndrome still did not exist, and "mongolism" continued to carry a powerful stigma of inherited "deficiency" or parental failing.

Doctors also would have assumed that a child such as Neil would be a continual source of disappointment and shame, further undermining the development of his siblings, who would struggle to cope with their family's identity as flawed or broken. The disabled child would therefore be shunned, to his or her own detriment. In the 1940s, doctors presented institutionalization as not only necessary "to preserve the 'normal' family," but also as preferable for the wellbeing of the disabled child.[14] Institutions would presumably provide some education and cultivate a sense of belonging and self-fulfillment, something the family would never be able to provide.

Most medical professionals at the time failed to recognize that bringing a child with Down syndrome into a family does not inherently overwhelm parents or tarnish the psychological development of siblings. Rather, it was the sheer lack of support systems—of accurate information and accessible services, or a broader tolerance of difference—that burdened caretakers and families. The systems that did exist in the 1940s, segregated institutions, were overcrowded and neglected, often run by incompetent staff who abused residents and did little to foster their wellbeing. And Erikson and Mead failed to anticipate that secretly institutionalizing Neil would become a source of lifelong despair for his siblings, the guilt of abandoning their brother far worse than any perceived stigma associated with his disability.

After Neil's birth, Erikson further developed his famous analysis of "normal" life cycle development, all while his disabled son remained hidden. Rather than protect the family, however, Neil's absence threatened to rip them apart.

.   .   .

After Neil's birth, Mead's views about disability and its impact on family life began to evolve. Over the 1950s, Mead would rise to the height of her own celebrity: she was viewed not only as an expert on childhood and psychological development across cultures, but also as a kind of national oracle, a sage commentator on changes in American life. She became a noted public figure, routinely invited to speak at academic conferences and to testify at government committees. She was also frequently sought out for media interviews. In addition to writing for popular magazines such as *Redbook* and *Ladies' Home Journal,* she appeared on television shows like *The Tonight Show* with Johnny Carson. *Time* magazine listed her in 1970 as one of the most influential people in the world.[15]

By the early 1950s, Mead found herself addressing parent groups that were challenging the logic of institutionalization and the assumption that children like Neil could not be cared for at home. Such parent advocacy groups were a recent phenomenon in American society. President Roosevelt's New Deal program in the late 1930s had emphasized a new role for the state in ensuring the social welfare of citizens, prompting the formation of civic groups claiming rights or resources. The aftermath of World War II also spurred a growing discourse of universal human rights. The UN charter was established in 1945 and the Universal Declaration of Human Rights was published three years later, powerfully asserting the idea of inherent human dignity and potential. Influenced by the expansion of the Civil Rights movement in the United States in the 1950s, parents increasingly asserted the rights of their disabled children and their entitlement to societal resources and government support.

The first parent groups that formed in the 1930s typically consisted of parents whose children were already living in institutions. These parents tended to view themselves as allies of institutions, not adversaries.[16] Not only did doctors recommend separating the disabled child from the family, but also officials discouraged parents from maintaining close bonds with children once they were institutionalized. Early parent groups challenged this, sometimes organizing visitations and social events, in addition to raising awareness and resources to improve institutional care. These groups also nurtured a sense of fellowship among parents of disabled children, drawing in parents who didn't or couldn't institutionalize their children. Although medical doctors routinely recommended institutionalization, especially of newborns with identifiable conditions, space was often limited and overcrowding was a chronic problem, leaving many parents no choice but to care for their disabled child.[17] Growing awareness over the 1940s and 1950s of overcrowding and abuse in institutions also motivated parents to keep their children at home.

But many felt isolated, their children neglected by medical professionals. Lacking useful advice from doctors and other professionals, parents turned to each other. One mother in New York City placed an announcement in a newspaper describing her son and asking to connect with other parents: "Surely there must be other children like him, other parents like myself. Where are you? Let's band together and do something for our children!" After other parents responded, they formed the local Association for the Help of Retarded Children (AHRC).[18] Parent groups such as the AHRC embraced the growing public discourse of universal human worth and dignity in justifying their formation and eventually in advocating for access to services in their communities and homes.

The first memoirs by parents describing their experiences of having a disabled child began to appear in the 1950s, contributing to growing public awareness and feelings of shared struggle. The prolific novelist Pearl S. Buck, a best-selling author in the 1930s who had won both the Pulitzer and Nobel prizes, wrote about her experiences with her disabled daughter in *The Child Who Never Grew*, first published in *Ladies' Home Journal* in 1950 and excerpted in both *Reader's Digest* and *Time*.[19] Buck was the daughter of missionaries who had raised her in China, and she spent much of her life before 1935 between China and the United States. In *The Child Who Never Grew*, Buck tells the story of realizing that her daughter Carol, born in 1920, was developmentally disabled. She pushes back against the eugenics-era assertion that feeblemindedness or mental deficiency stems from "tainted lineage" within the family.[20] She also challenges stigmas that associate disability with perversion or crime, drawing on the image of Carol as an "eternal child," innocent and joyful, and therefore deserving of love.

Medical doctors in the 1920s had little insight to offer Buck and her daughter was excluded from school, so Buck made the difficult decision to place her in an institution for her continued care. She recounts searching for an institution in the United States as a "stranger" in her own country, a cultural outsider longing to find a place that would acknowledge the "human quality" of her daughter.[21] She was disturbed by the "abode of horror" she found in some, where residents were "herded together like dogs."[22] When she finally placed nine-year-old Carol at the Training School at Vineland, New Jersey, she continued to visit her regularly. She emphasizes the importance of keeping Carol at home as long as she could and then maintaining a close relationship with her after institutionalization.

Buck portrayed children like her daughter as having inherent value. "Remember, too," wrote Buck, "that the child has his right to life, whatever that life may be, and he has the right to happiness, which you must find for him. Be proud of your child, accept him as he is and do not heed the words and stares of those who know no better. This child has a meaning for you and for all children."[23]

Buck's account was groundbreaking in the ways it challenged eugenics-era stigmas and contributed to a rising critique of institutions. It was soon followed by other memoirs, such as John Frank's *My Son's Story* in 1952, about his son Petey, who began to display developmental disabilities and have seizures as a toddler. Frank similarly presents Petey as fully human and emphasizes his being a part of their family even after they decide to place him in an institution for care.[24]

A year later, *Angel Unaware* by Dale Evans Rogers became a bestseller. Evans and her singing cowboy husband, Roy Rogers, were already celebrities when the book was published and they would go on to star together in dozens of movies and TV shows, release hundreds of recordings, and tour around the world. Their daughter, Robin, was born with Down syndrome in 1950 and died as a two-year-old from complications of mumps. *Angel Unaware* is an inspirational story written from Robin's perspective "as an angel in heaven recounting to God her brief experiences on earth," emphasizing the beauty of Robin's humanity, her inherent innocence and virtue, and how her brief life transformed others around her.[25] The response to the already famous Dale Evans Rogers and Roy Rogers was an outpouring of public sympathy.

Parent memoirs such as these often relied on simplistic stereotypes of people with disabilities as angelic and eternal children. Used to humanize disabled children in the wake of the eugenics era, such stereotypes still circulate today in condescending ways that diminish the rights and personhood of people with disabilities, contributing to low expectations and reinforcing an association of disability with lack of autonomy.[26] Early parent memoirs, however, also asserted the inherent dignity of children with disabilities and drew attention to a reality experienced by many families in the United States. Parents struggled to care for their children at home without adequate information or support, and they agonized over the advice to institutionalize their children. Pearl Buck wrote in 1950 of often being asked to meet with "parents' organizations, parents of mentally deficient children who are coming together in their deep need for mutual comfort and support. Most of them are young people, and how my heart aches for them!"[27]

Mead, too, was increasingly asked to meet with such organizations, drawn into an emerging parent advocacy movement. Mead spoke on "Learning from the Handicapped" in 1950 at the annual meeting of the Handicapped Children's Home Service, an organization based in New York that coordinated volunteers to provide home-based recreational and educational services to children with disabilities. In 1954, she addressed the annual convention of the National Society for Crippled Children and Adults, an organization originally founded in 1919 with a focus on children and now known as Easterseals. A newspaper report describes her as emphasizing the theme of "triumph over circumstances, rather than the elements of pitifulness and dependence." It reports her saying that "the handicapped person must use one sense rather than another, approach the world from a different angle, rely on a different part of his body for dealing with the world around him and interacting with other people." This perspective, the experience of disability, enriches our "whole understanding of human behavior."[28]

Few, if any, anthropologists talked about disability as something enriching, as an aspect of the human experience worth understanding. In a 1959 televised interview, Mead elaborated further. "As our medical knowledge increases," asked the interviewer in an echo of eugenic fears from previous decades, "does this mean that we're going to have more and more people but of second-rate caliber?"

"I think we are going to have to widen the range of people who we treat as human," responded Mead. "And we build our society so they can live in it, so the deaf can live in it, the blind can live in it, and people with special disabilities. At the same time, we may hope to have a greater range of human variability, and therefore greater ability also."[29]

That same year, Mead was featured as a keynote speaker by the American Association on Mental Deficiency (AAMD), now called the American

Association on Intellectual and Developmental Disabilities. The AAMD was founded in 1876 as the Association of Medical Officers of American Institutions for Idiotic and Feebleminded Persons; its name changed multiple times over the century in response to evolving understandings of intellectual disability. Even though she was an anthropologist, Mead had numerous connections to the fields of psychology and mental health. Since the 1930s, she had maintained close professional ties with Erik Erikson and other prominent psychological researchers. During World War II, she was also involved in analyzing behavioral and cultural traits as part of national character studies, which purported to decode a shared public psyche, joining Gregory Bateson and other anthropologists as part of an effort to increase morale at home and facilitate intercultural understanding as Americans fought abroad. Over subsequent decades, she maintained ties with various government agencies and other policy initiatives broadly related to mental health, at one point declining an invitation to serve as Secretary of Health, Education, and Welfare for President Lyndon Johnson, yet still advising him on women's issues.[30] In 1956, she served as the president of the World Federation for Mental Health, an international advocacy organization founded in 1948, the same year the World Health Organization was formed. She was also teaching at the Menninger Foundation in 1959, a famous school of psychiatry and a clinic then located in Topeka, Kansas. Mead had lectured there in the early 1940s and maintained an association with the Menninger Foundation for the rest of her career.

Mead was invited by the AAMD to offer an anthropological perspective at a symposium on "research design and methodology in mental retardation," hosted by the Woods Schools, a private institution in Langhorne, Pennsylvania.[31] In the 1950s, the AAMD, long a professional organization associated with institutionalization, found itself responding to broader social changes that drew into question its mission. Parents were increasingly questioning the need to segregate and confine their children with disabilities. Critique was also taking shape from within the ranks of experts. In 1942, for example, child psychiatrist Leo Kanner, today known as one of the first to identify the condition now called autism spectrum disorder, published the article "Exoneration of the Feebleminded," in which he criticized how societal prejudice burdens the intellectually disabled with a "double handicap"—disabilities from birth plus the crushing weight of social exclusion.[32] Basic terminology and assumptions were being questioned from within the profession.

In the late 1940s, some members of the AAMD started promoting the nascent parent's movement, welcoming their advocacy within the professional ranks. Annual conventions of the AAMD began dedicating time to advocacy, with local chapters of parent groups often in attendance. By 1949, some were calling to formally include parent-led advocacy groups within the AAMD. Incoming president Mildred Thompson insisted that the AAMD could more effectively support the parent movement by helping them create their own vehicle for organizing, and the following year a national conference for parents was held in Minneapolis, where Thompson worked as a state official.[33] The National Association of Parents and Friends of Retarded Children was officially chartered in 1953 and grew rapidly, drawing in thousands of parent groups from across the United States. Its name was changed in the 1970s to the National Association for Retarded Citizens (NARC), and in the 1990s simply to The Arc. Mead is said to have referred to The Arc as "the most effective voluntary action group in the country."[34]

Parent advocacy groups raised questions about the purpose of confinement, some advocating for home-based services and access to education in their communities. Others advocated for improving conditions and resources at public institutions. This split meant that organizations such as The Arc took a middle road in the 1950s, supporting parents who chose to raise a disabled child at home and lobbying to improve institutional conditions. This division played out among the AAMD membership as well. In 1954, a year after The Arc's founding, Arthur Hopwood, then the president of the AAMD, emphasized that "medicine, not education, will find the answers," insisting that investment in research should take priority over allocating resources for services that might improve the lives of children.[35]

Many professionals continued to view institutions as the appropriate destination for children with disabilities and maintained that only the "highest functioning" of disabled children were even capable of learning, and then only in the context of segregated education. In 1958, AAMD president Chris DeProspo refuted calls to make public education available to children with intellectual disabilities, suggesting instead that their learning should be limited to "arts and crafts" to "help them enjoy a life of conformity" in the context of "kindly institutional tutelage."[36]

Against this backdrop, Mead was invited to speak on a curious topic— "Research: Cult or Cure?"—which she interpreted in terms of how Americans, in their unique, culturally specific ways, perceive behavioral research. She used the opportunity to provide advice to professionals in the audience on how to better advocate for more resources for and recognition of their work with the "mentally deficient," or those diagnosed with what had only recently begun to be known as "mental retardation." She also interpreted this theme in terms of how an anthropological perspective might inform research in this field.

This entailed, for Mead, taking apart the idea of "mentally deficient" altogether, and roundly questioning the practice of institutionalization.

.   .   .   .   .   .

Mead stood at the podium, only to find that the microphone was far too tall for her. Organizers scrambled to lower it as she playfully scolded her hosts.[37] Barely over five feet tall, Mead nonetheless had an imposing presence, flashes of grey forming in her short, dark hair. Round glasses over wide eyes, she gazed steadily at her audience, now and then bringing her chin down to her chest to look over the frame of her glasses. She gave her presentation without notes, using a conversational style and frequently gesturing with her hands.

"I have been brought to my early youth by way of the recent monograph by Gladwin and Sarason," she began.[38]

Mead was known to disarm her audiences with sarcasm, and she began by mentioning an ambitious review of scholarly research published a year earlier, titled *Mental Subnormality: Biological, Psychological, and Cultural Factors*. The review, published in multiple outlets, was sponsored by the National Association of Retarded Children, and included anthropologist Thomas Gladwin among its authors.[39] He was sitting in the front row.

"I feel as if I have come full circle," she said wryly, noting she had received her master's degree in psychology for her 1926 study on language and intelligence testing, which was cited in the review. "This was a psychological study," she scoffed. "Therefore, it gets into the bibliography."

"Since then, I have been working in what is called cultural anthropology," she continued. She was a prolific writer and widely read by the public, but sometimes ignored by her professional colleagues. "So, nothing I have written gets into the bibliography."

Her folksy, engaging speaking style was captivating but also provocative. She mentioned, quite pointedly, that she had also reviewed the latest edition of a standard resource in the field, A. F. Tredgold's *Textbook of Mental Deficiency*, originally published in 1908. This was a barb aimed directly at the professionals in the audience. Tredgold supported eugenics and described euthanasia as a remedy to relieve society's burden of caring for mentally defective groups. His son, R. F. Tredgold, had helped edit the latest edition, referenced by Mead, following in his father's footsteps and retaining the suggestion of mass murder to manage the feebleminded.[40] Wolf Wolfensberger, who would help revolutionize the profession in the 1970s, recalled how the enduring hold of the Tredgold textbook revealed "the poverty of our field in the 1950s."[41] Mead was reminding her audience of their profession's dangerous legacy.

"Since I have been asked to come back into the fold and give this talk this morning," she continued, "I myself am a demonstration of many of the points that the Gladwin and Sarason monograph makes—that people are not paying enough attention; that we haven't been focusing adequately on the problem of mental retardation; that we have put it in a box; that we have put the children whom we so classify in separate institutions and have forgotten them."[42]

In their monograph, Sarason and Gladwin summarized a growing body of cross-cultural research that drew into question the very categories of "normality" and "abnormality," the very terms used to talk about and respond to disability. "Even a child with a severe defect," they wrote, "must be viewed as deficient *relative to* cultural standards of acceptability; the cause of his deficiency may be organic, but its magnitude is dependent upon social criteria."[43] As anthropologist Marvin Opler explained in a 1959 review, "the concept of normality is at best a statistical construct. And the important issue, now as always, is to learn more about the continuum of human development."[44] Accounts of so-called mental retardation in other cultures often found very different attitudes and systems of classification, systems in which such conditions were often unremarkable.[45]

"If we really studied the children we are classifying today as mentally retarded," Mead explained, "children we are excluding from attention, putting in institutions, and giving up as hopeless, if we really studied them properly and took into account the factors that we know all about now—the effect of educational deprivation, of emotional deprivation—showed how this went with social discrimination, with bad housing, with low economic level, it would show up conditions in our society that we don't want to face."

By "show up," Mead meant it would reveal the social conditions that shaped the experiences of disability and the quality of life of people with disabilities. Mead focused on the social and economic conditions that made raising a disabled child at home difficult and that limited the potential of such children, much as she had in her concerns about the challenges facing families in industrial society. She continued, "It would show up how bad our school system is, how bad our IQ tests are, how unimaginative our whole educational system is—narrow, meager, dull, and so forth."[46] We've known for decades, she said, that what we try to "measure" through IQ is actually "diversified," with different people having "different kinds of intelligence."

"We took all this study of difference and put it in a single scale," creating categories of abnormality. Then we "cut off the mentally retarded, put them in a box, treat them as a separate problem, as hopeless, irreversible, not really worth too much attention."[47]

The "box," for Mead, was certainly both figurative and literal. She was talking about abstract, conceptual categories such as "feebleminded" and "mental deficient" and "retarded," categories of abnormality filled with meaning through the flawed logics of intelligence tests and the cultural imperatives of modern schools, which rank children through grading systems and tacitly encourage competition, as if a pupil's success or failure stems from individual merit alone. "Boxes" were also the actual institutions and schools for the feebleminded, the places where children such as Neil Erikson were sent at birth, then neglected and eventually forgotten.

Mead, of course, was not the first to critique institutions. Parent advocacy groups spotlighted the conditions and quality of institutions, and several high-profile exposés were published in the 1940s. Albert Maisel's article "Bedlam 1946" for *Life* magazine examined the horrendous conditions of psychiatric institutions and was accompanied by dozens of disturbing photos. "The vast majority of our state mental institutions," he wrote, "are dreary, dilapidated excuses for hospitals, costly monuments to the states' betrayal of the duty they have assumed to their most helpless wards."[48] Channing Richardson published "A Hundred Thousand Defectives" that same year in *Christian Century*, also criticizing institutionalization.[49] Mary Jane Ward's 1947 semi-autobiographical novel *The Snake Pit*, about a woman's recovery from mental illness and experience in a psychiatric hospital, was made into an Oscar-winning film a year after publication. Exposés such as Frank Leon Wright's 1947 *Out of Sight, Out of Mind* provided another insider account as part of a growing movement for change. Journalist Albert Deutsch published *Shame of the States* in 1948, an influential social history that called for broad reform. Many of his informants included conscientious objectors to World War II who were assigned service in state psychiatric institutions, but whose sense of social justice led them to speak out about overcrowding and abuse.

Despite calls for reform, the number of people living in institutional settings grew over the 1950s and 1960s. Some had assumed the problems described in the exposés had stemmed from a lack of adequate funding or other resources.[50] But overcrowding and abusive treatment continued even when funding improved. In 1965, Robert Kennedy toured the Willowbrook State School in New York, which he described to the national media as a dehumanizing snake pit. Several months later, the 1966 essay *Christmas in Purgatory*, by Burton Blatt and Fred Kaplan, used hundreds of covertly taken photographs to bring readers into the back halls of several institutions, exposing "naked patients groveling in their own feces, children in locked cells, horribly crowded dormitories, and understaffed and wrongly staffed facilities."[51] They described an overwhelming stench of human excretions, naked bodies curled on the floor as other residents mingled above them, the relentless sounds of moaning, of despair. They found children's dormitories with dozens of kids locked into rooms, desperate for interaction, "lying, rocking, sleeping, sitting," some banging their heads against walls, blood spilling from split foreheads.[52] Several years later, Americans encountered such dreadful scenes in their living rooms with Geraldo Rivera's 1972 investigative report, the thirty-minute documentary *Willowbrook: The Last Great Disgrace*. He recorded the striking scenes and unforgettable "mournful wail" of neglected children and described the horrendous odor in horrid terms: "it smelled of filth, it smelled of disease, it smelled of death." The public outrage that followed helped galvanize a push to reform or close such institutions.[53]

Institutions became the subject of sociological interest in the 1960s with Erving Goffman's now famous work on stigma. In 1961, he published *Asylums,* a series of four essays that expounded on the concept of the "total institution," places where inmates are stripped of a previous identity and inscribed with a new one as part of their conscription. Such institutions solidify rigid roles and categories of identity, routinizing them as if they are preexisting rather than imposed by society, creating the very pathologies they purport to treat. Mead, it turns out, was already familiar with Goffman's work when she addressed the AAMD in 1959, having gotten a preview a few years earlier. As Goffman was developing the famous essays that would appear in *Asylums,* he presented his idea of the total institution at a 1956 conference on "group processes" sponsored by the Josiah Macy Jr. Foundation.[54] Mead was in the audience, along with her friend and ex-husband Gregory Bateson. Both Mead and Bateson engaged in several substantive exchanges with Goffman as the young scholar attempted to present his ideas.

At the AAMD podium, Mead paused, peering over her glasses at her audience, a group of experts who still largely defined their profession in terms of institutions that confined people categorized as "abnormal." The very basis of their profession was culturally arbitrary and harmful to the children they claimed to be helping, she was trying to tell them. If we are to research people defined as "mentally deficient," she said, the focus should not be on trying to "cure" their conditions, but on learning from them so that we can make society more accommodating. She spoke of increasing our understanding for the purpose of "adapting the world to the people," to "build a culture in which they belong."[55] We should shape the world to fit the children, she said. The goal should be to bring more people "into the possibility of learning."[56]

To illustrate, Mead then told a story about a "little mongoloid girl" who had been diagnosed at a young age. The girl, said Mead, was now in her teenage years. *Neil Erikson would have been fifteen years old at the time, still alive in an institution, rarely visited by his parents. His siblings knew of his existence by now, but never visited him, and assumed they were supposed to pretend that he had never been born.*

"She was given every possibility that money and science could give at the period when she was born," continued Mead, "quite well tested and evaluated."[57]

Mead indicated that the girl's development had stagnated within the established models of care. A family member suggested they enroll the child at a local Catholic school. Mead offered few specifics and implied that the girl went to school and participated in other activities associated with the Catholic Church, such as being baptized and confirmed. But this wasn't about religion, Mead emphasized. The girl was included, allowed to participate in everyday community settings.

"She became a human being in a way that she had not been one before," explained Mead. She was acknowledged and valued as a whole person. She was seen for her potential, not for her deficits. "I think that what happened on the secular and human side with this little girl—was that for the first time she met a situation where people were willing to teach her the whole instead of saying, 'You are defective and you can only learn a part.'"[58]

"When I say that she became a human being, there is no doubt that she had a big deficit in ability to learn and to carry things through. But she became responsible; she became someone who could act in emergencies with responsibility. It didn't mean she could write books, but that is not the only definition of a human being."[59]

In addition to accepting diverse ways of being human, Mead emphasized the importance of learning from that diversity, of acknowledging what diverse minds and bodies contribute to the grand human experiment. "If we can recognize that to the extent that we understand better every child born into our society in any spot, and the way in which they learn and the way in which their minds work at different ages in different contexts, faced with different situations, we enrich not only the lives of those children, but our whole understanding of our culture."[60]

The published transcript of Mead's presentation includes two questions from the audience, which give some insight into how her comments were received. The questioners were skeptical, to put it mildly. One audience member pushed back against "the kind of perceptual revolution we should undergo in regard to mental defectives as not really defective, but people who in some way can change to normal people by recognizing that they have something to give us."

It's not about making "everybody normal," Mead countered. We are "not hunting for one kind of mind ... What I said was that we could make many, many more people parts of the whole, functioning human beings ... a full representative of their culture."

"It is quite plain, Dr. Mead, from the comments you have made," said another audience member, "that you have some sizable dissatisfaction with the American culture and the way in which it is handling this problem. I wonder if you could give us some guide, as an anthropologist, as to what cultures you are familiar with that we could pattern ourselves after to help reach the ideal that you are looking for."

"The fact that people can be dissatisfied with the American culture is one of its virtues," responded Mead. "And I haven't any desire for us to pattern ourselves after anybody. What I have a desire for is for us to learn by the analysis of other cultures things that we could do and want to do."

.   .   .   .   .

Margaret Mead wasn't calling for a "perceptual revolution." She was describing an actual revolution, driven partly by parents but increasingly also by disabled self-advocates.[61] Mead's own perspective on disability grew as she participated in this movement, called upon as an open-minded, progressive expert on human development. In 1944 she had been an accomplice in sending Neil Erikson to an institution, perhaps thinking she was helping to protect the Erikson family. Twenty years later, the year before Neil died, Mead wrote a preface to *You Can Raise Your Handicapped Child*, written by Evelyn West Ayrault, a psychologist with cerebral palsy who authored the book to help empower parents to keep their families together. Mead describes Ayrault in 1964 as a new type of "specialist in helping others," akin to a medical doctor or other helping profession practitioner, a category taking shape "from among those with a given problem" or disability, those who combine personal experience with professional training for the benefit of others. "It is her own life that says to the parents of handicapped children—and to the children themselves," wrote Mead, "*It can be done.*"[62]

Writers and self-advocates such as Ayrault sought not only to help parents navigate the challenges of raising a child with a disability, but also to identify potential resources and services. New vocational rehabilitation programs and services took shape in the post-World War II period as government policy responded to the needs of disabled veterans reintegrating into society.[63] The frequency of workplace accidents in industrial America also meant disability would become an important issue for the labor movement as it sought to secure and expand the rights of workers.[64] For parents raising children with disabilities, an array of programs and services slowly became available in the communities where they lived, as did new tools for asserting the rights of their children as they fought to help them become contributing members of society. Many parents, however, lacked basic information about what services they might try to access. They also confronted beliefs and attitudes suggesting such services should be directed toward making people with disabilities into "productive" citizens, implying that one's worth is defined only in terms of the ability to work and contribute economically. If a child lacked the intellectual or physical abilities to become productive—to work, to earn a living, to contribute economically, to operate as a cog in the wealth accumulation machine—then there was no point in investing resources into their development, no point in including them in society.

Mead challenged this attitude during a keynote address to the 1967 meeting of the President's Committee on Employment of the Handicapped, which had been created by President Eisenhower a decade earlier and would become the Office of Disability Employment Policy in 2001. With roughly three thousand people in attendance, she spoke perched atop a suitcase so that she could be seen over the podium and its cluster of microphones, part of a keynote lineup that included Vice President Hubert Humphrey. By this point in her career, Mead's public persona often featured her wearing a long, dark cape and using a tall, forked walking stick, which she brought with her to the podium as she propped herself on the suitcase. She began with an anecdote about scientists who had discovered human fossils that showed evidence of a fractured bone that had healed. In the long arc of human evolution, "we know we are approaching what we regard as true humanity" when we encounter the trace of someone who had been disabled by injury and who would have most certainly starved to death if not "cared for by the other members of the group."[65] Progress, said Mead, is measured by people's ability to recognize their shared humanity, to provide care even for "any infant who showed any deviation from the norm."[66]

Mead then suggested moving beyond a focus on the seeming "deficiencies" of people with disabilities. "We are too fixated on the notion that if we can only equip every handicapped person to function as if they were like other people," said Mead, "that is enough. I don't think that is enough."[67] Instead, she asked the audience to consider what people with disabilities contribute in a broad, holistic sense, expanding "our humanity" and "our imagination," deepening "our understanding of the world."[68]

Although commonly ignored or overlooked, disability is rather commonplace. Even if we consider ourselves able-bodied now, we will all become disabled at some point, whether due to injury, sickness, or simply because of the aging process. "I have spent quite a little time in a wheelchair with a bad ankle," explained Mead, who had first broken her right ankle in 1924 when she was hit by a taxicab in New York City. She broke it again in 1929 during fieldwork in Manus, Papua New Guinea, and was treated by a local bonesetter. When Mead conducted fieldwork among the Arapesh in 1931 with her then-husband Reo Fortune, she was transported to a mountaintop village "strapped like a pig to a carrying pole," and was stranded when the people hired to carry her and their belongings refused to go any further.[69] She broke the same ankle again in 1960 and then started using a cane, the distinctive forked staff that many assumed was part of her persona as a venerable public seer.

"I use it because I have a bad ankle," conceded Mead. "No one associates my stick with a handicap because it is so peculiar."[70]

As she had begun doing in the 1950s, Mead talked about disability not as something in need of fixing or changing, but as a basic human reality worthy of anthropological attention. "Every person with a handicap of any sort lives in a world inaccessible to other people," she explained. For anthropologists, the challenge is how to gain access to this world, in the same way that an anthropologist like Mead worked to gain access to the distinct cultural worlds of the Manus or Arapesh. The Arapesh, for instance, whom Mead described as gentle and cooperative in her analysis of how culture shapes the meaning and enactment of gender, don't just speak different languages, or have different beliefs. They inhabit and experience different cultural worlds. For Mead, fieldwork involved trying to get as close as possible to that *other* experience, then describing it in terms intelligible to her American audiences. This entailed attempting to learn a new language and develop rapport with locals, participating in everyday life to see things from their perspective. These are acts of translation, the anthropologist moving between the internalized beliefs and values of their own culture and the ones they are trying to document and understand.

To illustrate, Mead briefly described the research of her student, John Langston Gwaltney, who had defended his dissertation just the day before. Born in 1928, Gwaltney had lost his vision soon after birth and was the first blind student to attend his high school in New Jersey. Later in his career, when he was a professor at Syracuse University, he would become known for his 1980 book *Drylongso: A Self-Portrait of Black America*, the work of a Black anthropologist using ethnography to document the lived experiences and struggles of other Black people in the United States. It was widely acclaimed outside the discipline and viewed by other anthropologists as an early example of what was once known as "native anthropology" or turning the anthropological gaze on oneself and one's own culture.[71] After graduating from Upsala College in 1952, Gwaltney went on to complete a master's degree in 1957 from the New School for Social Research (Mead taught courses there from 1954 until 1978). He then pursued his PhD in anthropology from Columbia University, supervised by Mead.

For his PhD research, at a time when anthropologists were still expected to study "exotic" cultures, Gwaltney conducted fieldwork in 1963 and 1964 among the Chinantec-speakers of San Pedro Yólox, a settlement of subsistence farmers in the rugged highlands of Oaxaca, Mexico. In the 1960s, this community had extraordinarily high rates of a disease called onchocerciasis. Known as river blindness, the disease is caused by infection with a parasitic worm spread by biting flies. The flies propagate along riverbanks and in the shady groves of coffee plantations in tropical regions of the world, biting people's exposed torsos, arms, necks, and faces as they bathe or work the fields, leaving larvae to develop in subcutaneous nodules. A parasite then makes its way into the bloodstream, eventually infecting ocular tissue and causing lesions that lead to progressive and irreversible loss of sight. In San Pedro Yólox, men descended from their village for decades to participate in seasonal agricultural work, exposing themselves to the flies. The condition became so pervasive and routinized that eventually blindness was an expected part of the aging process.[72] It wasn't until the mid-1980s that the antiparasitic drug Ivermectin became widely available, a single dose clearing the body of worms for several months and preventing disease onset. (Ivermectin was, coincidently, the same drug promoted by conspiracy theorists and antivaccine activists as a miracle cure for COVID-19 at the height of the pandemic.)

Funded by the National Institute of Mental Health, Gwaltney's research was truly unique at the time because he documented the experience of river blindness among ordinary people engaged in the mundane tasks of getting by while coping with socioeconomic inequalities.[73] He wanted to know what blindness meant to them, how they handled loss of vision, and how it impacted the larger community. As a Black and blind anthropologist, Gwaltney's work was also groundbreaking because he was able to access a world that Mead framed as inaccessible to those with sight, but that she had come to value as another laboratory of human behavior worthy of serious anthropological attention.

Most ethnographic fieldwork begins by visually mapping a site. In their books or other accounts of the research experience, many anthropologists first describe an arrival scene, a convention that illustrates how vision is widely taken for granted as a preeminent mode of "observation" in the social sciences.[74] Equipped with a braille typewriter and a tape recorder, Gwaltney mapped the community through other sensory modalities, starting with the "auditory rhythms of the pueblo." The sounds he encountered were initially unintelligible to him and "had to be explained by villagers who took them for granted."[75] This was complicated by the steep mountainous terrain and intense seasonal rains.

"The heavy summer and autumnal rains," he explains, "convert the precipitous tracks of the village into a network of diminutive torrents, each with a number of miniature cataracts. The several streams that flow through and around the village and the rest of the *municipio* are high from June to October. Traversing these watercourses or traveling anywhere near them imposes special difficulties upon any person who is obliged to hear his way, for they roar like heavy, sustained surf for at least half the year, obscuring and distorting all other sounds in their vicinity."[76]

He also found that his walking sticks were of limited use for independently navigating and feeling his way across the uneven, rocky terrain with its sharp, rutted slopes and the sometimes-unpredictable routes of wandering livestock.[77] As Mead recounted, "he noted that all of the children in this society have as a major part of their childhood, the function of serving as the eyes of the blind. No blind person is ever without a lively, interested child." Sighted children routinely assisted blind adults, not as a chore or out of pity, but as a deferential encounter with a community elder, chatting informally as they traversed the town, casually helping them navigate obstacles. "I had to learn to trust those children completely," Gwaltney told Mead. "Unless I could trust them completely, they couldn't lead me safely and I would land in the river."

The world Gwaltney found contrasted sharply with his own experiences in the United States.[78] Yoleño children, he says, "are accustomed to seeing blind persons from earliest youth" and don't display the "reactions of fear, hostility and ridicule that blind persons often encounter in North American children." They have "always known that some people perceive the world without sight" and "expressed surprise when asked why they acted as guides, assuming children everywhere performed this service." While river blindness was experienced as loss and suffering, Gwaltney also interpreted blindness in this community as "the agent of a rare transgenerational empathy." The ways sighted adults and children support those with river blindness helps "forge a greater degree of communal solidarity by binding the very old and the very young together with ties of service, affection and never-failing tact. Despite their special problems, the Yoleño blind are not marginal."[79]

Disability is a social phenomenon in Gwaltney's accounts, given meaning within the context of people's lives, their connections to family, their role in a community. Though their blindness results from a nasty disease that accompanies other collective traumas (ranging from natural disasters and economic exploitation to political violence) shaping the lives of subsistence farmers in southern Mexico, it is not *only an affliction,* and it is not *only an individual's impairment.* Rather, it's a shared challenge—an impairment, yes, but also simultaneously generative of something beneficial for the collective.

Mead, too, addressed the social significance of disability. Social conditions marginalize people with intellectual disabilities, limit their humanity, ignore their potential. These conditions can be changed. In her presentation to the President's Committee on Employment of the Handicapped, she emphasized that the changes occurring to provide opportunities to people with physical disabilities hinted at a more fundamental transformation.

"Every time a building is built with a ramp, people in wheelchairs can use it," said Mead. "But so can old ladies and old gentlemen and children who have just learned to walk. In a sense, this device for the handicapped has benefited all."[80]

In other words, Mead stressed that the goal should not be merely to foster economic productivity among the disabled, as if their worth were defined only by the rules of capitalism. Rather, the goal is to cultivate an ethic of caring for others, to cultivate inclusion and access because doing so is the basis of a fair and just society and acknowledges the basic truth that not all people perceive and experience the world in the same way.

There is something fundamentally human about disability.

.   .   .   .   .

Few anthropologists explored disability in the 1960s as a window into understanding the human condition, making Gwaltney's study of river blindness and Mead's public remarks about disability rather exceptional. Like Mead, anthropology would slowly be pushed into new directions by the broader disability rights movement. One of the first efforts to study the lives of people with intellectual disabilities through ethnography was Robert Edgerton's 1967 *The Cloak of Competence: Stigma in the Lives of the Mentally Retarded,* published just as critique of institutionalization was growing. His study documented the efforts of intellectually disabled adults to adapt to life outside of institutional care and confinement.

Mead's interest in child development and public policy related to children would keep her connected to the parent advocacy movement and the disability rights movement that unfolded in the 1970s. Even as Mead was dying from cancer in 1978, she continued working and writing, preparing notes for her regular column in *Redbook*. After her death in November of that year, her friend and collaborator Rhoda Métraux organized and edited Mead's notes on the International Year of the Child, which were published in May 1979 as "A Mother's Day Message: What We Can Do Now for Our Children's Future." The essay was wide-ranging, and in one section applauds changes taking place in the care of children with disabilities and calls for "schools that teach and teaching that will include handicapped children as full members of the school community."[81]

Full membership, in the sense not only of access and inclusion, but also of recognition as a person, has been a generational struggle that continues today. In the 1970s, major battles were taking place so that children with disabilities could simply go to school. Intellectual disability began to receive national attention a decade earlier following the election of John F. Kennedy and the advocacy of his wealthy, politically connected family. His sister, Rosemary, experienced seizures and struggled with learning as a child. When her behavior was said to become "erratic" as a young adult, she was treated with a frontal lobe lobotomy. In 1941, with Rosemary mildly sedated so that she could verbally respond to questions, doctors sliced into her skull, making small incisions on both sides of her forehead, then inserted an instrument reminiscent of a butter knife, gently moving it back and forth to sever brain tissue.

It was a horrendous failure, as most lobotomies were, leaving her mentally incapacitated, no longer able to walk or speak at twenty-three years old. Her family quietly placed Rosemary in a private institution in Jefferson, Wisconsin, where she lived the remainder of her life. While the procedure was kept secret for forty years, part of her story became widely known two decades later when John F. Kennedy's political rise provided a platform for his sister Eunice Kennedy Shriver, who would become a prominent advocate and a founder of the Special Olympics. "Mental retardation can happen in any family," wrote Shriver in 1962. "It has happened in the families of the poor and the rich, of governors, senators, Nobel prizewinners, doctors, lawyers, writers, men of genius, presidents of corporations—the president of the United States."[82]

After he became president in 1961, Kennedy created the President's Panel on Mental Retardation and supported the founding of the National Institute for Child Health and Human Development (NICHD), which emphasized expanding basic research on the causes and circumstances of intellectual disability.[83] As such research programs expanded, Mead found herself providing testimony, sometimes alongside advocates from The Arc, about the complex and multifaceted causes of intellectual disability, and the need for federally supported research on human development. No society, she told the Joint Commission on Mental Health of Children in 1969, "can strive to do anything less than make maximum use of all its human potential, and to stop the tragic waste of human potential which is occurring today."[84]

The language of human development and unrecognized potential, increasingly used by Mead and others, reflected a wider paradigm shift in the 1960s. Psychologists such as Edward Zigler, one of the architects of the federal Head Start program, argued against the once widely held view that children with intellectual disabilities were inherently different, suggesting instead that their development was slowed or impeded, affected by complex physical and social factors that needed to be better understood. Advocacy organizations embraced the new developmental model, contending that all children are capable of learning and development.[85]

Policy reforms also embraced the concept of normalization, initially advanced by Bengt Nirje, then head of the Swedish Parents Association for Retarded Children. He was invited to tour the United States and contribute a chapter to *Changing Patterns in Residential Services for the Mentally Retarded,* where he defined normalization as "making available to the mentally retarded patterns and conditions of everyday life, which are as close as possible to the norms and patterns of mainstream society."[86] Further developed by other psychologists such as Wolf Wolfensberger, normalization would become the calling card of institutional and policy reforms, emphasizing direct, small-scale services within community settings.[87]

For many parents, this meant having their children attend local schools. But parents commonly encountered resistance from school administrators or others who claimed that children with disabilities, especially cognitive or learning disabilities, burdened the school district with additional costs, siphoning resources from the so-called promising kids. It was the same logic that had been used to justify institutionalizing children like Neil Erikson: to raise them at home would harm the other children in the family; to include them at school would be unfair to the others. Struggles for racial justice and civil rights in the 1950s and 1960s, however, had fundamentally altered many American's understandings of basic rights and notions of equality, including those of parents advocating on behalf of their children. When, in *Brown v. Board of Education*, the U.S. Supreme Court rejected the claim that segregated schools or programs could be equal, it provided a new moral and legal standard to guide parent advocacy in relation to disability. Groups such as The Arc adopted the language of civil rights; in 1973 it changed its name from the National Association for Retarded Children to the National Association for Retarded Citizens. As courts and state legislatures increasingly asserted the right of all children to access a public education, the federal government finally passed the Education for All Handicapped Children Act in 1975, later renamed the Individuals with Disabilities Education Act (IDEA).

In the 1970s, other legislative reforms ensured that inclusion would come to be understood as a civil right, at least in the eyes of the law, even if true social acceptance and belonging remained another struggle entirely. In addition to IDEA, Section 504 of the 1973 Rehabilitation Act adopted language from the 1964 Civil Rights Act to prohibit discrimination based on disability in any program that receives federal funding. Section 504 received little attention when the 1973 act was passed but became the focus of disability rights activists. People with disabilities routinely faced employment discrimination and barriers to accessing public transportation, buildings, or other spaces such as university campuses. Through a combination of persistent advocacy and strategic direct action, such as demonstrations and the occupation of federal buildings in 1977, activists successfully challenged the federal government's reluctance to enforce the new policy. In conjunction with IDEA, Section 504 ensured that schools receiving federal funds could not deny students with disabilities a free and appropriate education and reinforced principles of inclusion and accommodation.[88]

"We are making some fresh beginnings," wrote Mead just before her death,

> based on better knowledge, in our methods of care for children with different kinds of handicaps. In the past, too many handicapped children could receive some education and training only by leaving their homes and living for months and years in special institutions, where they were cut off from play with well children and from the everyday life of a community of families, adults and children of all kinds. Legislation has been passed. But as yet how many children with handicaps have open to them both the special help they so urgently need and education in the company of other children? How many teachers are we training to carry this additional, complex educational load?[89]

.   .   .   .   .

Decades after Mead's death, similar principles and challenges still structure my own daughter's journey through the public educational system. Schools are required to be accessible and to provide accommodations to meet the unique needs of students with disabilities, expectations reinforced through the Americans with Disabilities Act (ADA) of 1990, which generally prohibits discrimination based on disability. That children with disabilities will attend school in their communities is now assumed, though parents still often find themselves fighting for meaningful accommodations to help their children learn and develop alongside their peers. An entire generation has come of age in a post-ADA era in which concepts such as accommodation and inclusion are official policy at educational institutions.[90]

"Inclusion," however, remains a murky idea and is not explicitly mandated by law.[91] Instead, court rulings have generally emphasized the requirement of a "free appropriate public education" in the "least restrictive environment," and schools are expected to provide "reasonable accommodations" to meet such goals. Concepts such as "least restrictive" and "reasonable" are subject to interpretation, meaning the experience of children may vary from one school to the next, depending on resources, training of teachers, institutional norms, and the level of engagement of parents in advocating for their children. To some extent, accommodating physical disabilities has been more straightforward, as it's possible to create and enforce uniform design standards to make buildings or other physical spaces accessible: curb cuts, ramps, elevators, doorways, et cetera. These sorts of accommodations are visible and, as Mead noted, benefit a wide range of people. Many buildings, though not all, have been retrofitted and new ones must meet building codes to comply with federal law. In contrast, accommodating cognitive disability or neurodiversity is a more challenging task, as it involves rethinking dominant modes of teaching and learning, becoming attuned to different ways of perceiving the world.

When I was in junior high and high school in the early 1990s, the shift to inclusive education that began decades earlier and gained momentum with passage of the ADA meant that students with cognitive disabilities were sometimes included in mainstream classes, but more often were segregated into "special education" classes in the same school. I have memories from junior high of one or two kids with disabilities joining the rest of us during physical education class and recess but remaining separated during other parts of the day. This sort of partial inclusion occurred in a social context where, as adolescents, we were becoming increasingly image-conscious and judgmental of others. We often viewed our disabled peers as a curiosity, as kids who were allowed to be with the rest of us during specific times. Little effort was made to reform the educational system itself to make all classrooms inclusive to a diverse range of bodies and minds, or to cultivate tolerance and appreciation for bodies and minds that appeared to us as out of the ordinary.

Even today, this often continues as the dominant model. Although children with disabilities are automatically included in mainstream educational environments, as with Michaela their inclusion is often facilitated by a parallel service-based system with symbolic boundaries that risk stigmatizing and separating such students as different. Many public schools lack adequate resources and are forced to pack students into classrooms, with the pedagogy geared toward standardized learning, uniform skills, and teaching to the test. "Inclusion" for children with disabilities means finding ways to plug them into the existing system, not rethinking the flaws of the system itself. A shadow system built around the administering of services such as speech therapy, occupational therapy, physical therapy, and special education functions in parallel with the dominant educational model.

When Michaela turned four years old, she transitioned from the county-run Birth-to-3 program to the area school district, which provided services through its prekindergarten or what in Wisconsin is called four-year-old kindergarten or 4k. This didn't really entail a significant change for her. She had been receiving speech and occupational therapies through a combination of Birth-to-3 and services covered by our health insurance. After Birth-to-3 ended, we met with school-based service providers to develop an individualized education plan, or IEP, as Michaela left one system and entered another. She continued to attend her daycare program and was visited weekly by speech and occupational therapists from the school district. When she started kindergarten, the plan was basically to include her in a regular class and see how she did, while periodically removing her from class for targeted speech therapy. The transition from 4k to kindergarten ended up being a substantial adjustment. Michaela had attended the 4k program at the daycare center on the university campus, which not only provided childcare but was also integrated into the undergraduate early childhood education program. Lead teachers often had advanced college degrees and training in special education. Each day was organized around a thoughtful play-based pedagogy. Teachers also supervised college students who worked and trained in the center, which translated into an impressive ratio of adults to kids in the room. The experience for Michaela was positive and fulfilling. It was a flexible, low-pressure environment, and she learned and made friends.

Elementary school was different. Even when Aidric first started school, we noticed a stronger emphasis on compliance to behavioral norms and expectations. With more students, fewer teachers, and a rigid schedule, schools aim to foster self-discipline and conformity. Aidric struggled with this during kindergarten and his teacher started emailing us within the first month of the school year, asking for thoughts about how to address his "behavioral problems." We were shocked. She described attention issues that we had never ourselves witnessed or found concerning and she complained about him goofing off with other kids, things we always felt reflected his curious and playful demeanor. I told her it sounded like he was bored. Michaela, too, had a tricky transition to kindergarten. Within weeks it was clear that she struggled to stay on task and comply with the norms of the classroom.

But in contrast to the preschool environment, the school operates in a model where only students like Michaela are viewed as having unique needs. They hired a paraprofessional to support her in the classroom and throughout the day. This was a tremendous help but was also revealing. Such support staff are usually the least educated and lowest paid but spend the most time with your child. In Wisconsin, they might have only a high school diploma and on average are paid only fourteen dollars an hour. They assist the classroom lead teacher and the other special education teachers, but their knowledge and experience working with children with different conditions inevitably varies tremendously.

We soon experienced firsthand what it means to include children like Michaela through a service-based system that accommodates children with disabilities but remains grounded in a logic of segregated abilities. Midway through Michaela's kindergarten year, a school psychologist requested to evaluate Michaela to update the designation on her IEP that makes her eligible for accommodations and is necessary to secure state and federal financial support. When she entered 4K, she had been eligible under the category of "Other Health Impairment" due to her Down syndrome diagnosis. The school psychologist wanted to update the designation to "Intellectual Disability."

A couple months later, Tiffani and I met with the IEP team on a weekday afternoon. The school was following numerous COVID-19 pandemic protocols and the meeting was held virtually. I scrambled to pick up Aidric and Michaela in time and then run home to get on my computer for the online meeting. Tiffani was attending the meeting from work, and I joined ten minutes late. When I finally signed on, I found the school psychologist summarizing the results of a series of competency tests, contemporary versions of intelligence testing. She had not sent us a copy of her results ahead of time and merely shared the document on the videocall screen as she scrolled through the preliminary report. It was a gut-wrenching series of scores and scales that purportedly demonstrated Michaela's wide range of deficiencies across almost all areas of learning and development. It was my understanding that the scales were based on comparison with her "typically developing" peers, but it seemed like a mass of evidence intended to "show" she was struggling. Various tables consistently described her as "below average" and "very low" and "extremely low," routinely placed her below the third percentile, sometimes "less than 0.1." What does that even mean, I thought?

Midway through the verbal pummeling I interjected to apologize for being late and to ask what the goal of the meeting was. The school psychologist became defensive and struggled to articulate a clear response. The symbolic carnage then continued as she scrolled through the report and the evidence amassed to demonstrate Michaela's "below average" performance. I interjected again to say I could read the numbers myself and it wasn't necessary to list them off systemically. Instead, I asked to discuss how the results would help us understand how Michaela learns or guide how we make accommodations to maximize her potential. Silence. She was not thinking about this. The IEP team was not prepared to discuss this. This was just an obligatory meeting to convey test results focused on measuring, on producing a systematic accounting of Michaela's "deficits," rendered in numbers, displayed in scales, compared to "averages"—the euphemisms for normality.

We learned a difficult lesson that day about "accommodation" and "inclusion." Yes, it's true that Michaela is lucky to be born in an era in which it is simply assumed she will attend school in her community with her peers, and in which an entire system is set up to ensure she receives the accommodations she needs to fully participate, to learn, to achieve her potential. She has clearly benefited from various community-based support programs that were set into motion for her from the day she was born. We did not have to search for this or fight for this. It was already in place, the fruits of previous generations of parents, of advocates, of reformers who changed the world. I am truly thankful for the wonderful, thoughtful, caring people who have worked with Michaela and who will undoubtedly be a part of her life in the future.

But this system, for all the good things it enables, also perpetuates some fundamental problems. The service-based system, with the morass of paperwork and rules that trigger access to resources to pay for specialists to assist Michaela at school, obligates us to participate in an utterly demeaning process, one built around documenting and ranking the significance of Michaela's abilities. This process forces people into a belittling categorical mode of thinking that emphasizes inherent weaknesses.[92] It is also grounded in a deeply rooted contradiction: accommodating and including in practice, but then segregating in spirit, in attitude, in expectation. The logic of intelligence testing and psychological assessments is one that fails to acknowledge Michaela as a whole person, one that ignores her forms of intelligence, her way of perceiving the world.

I recognize that such assessments may be useful tools under the right circumstances. But these tools carry a century of ideological baggage and risk harming as well as helping. Under the current system, Michaela is included to the extent that additional services are delivered in parallel to a world from which she is symbolically excluded. The silence that followed my question about how the assessment results would help us understand the ways Michaela learns was revealing. The assessment was being used instead to determine her ability to conform. But to what extent will it penalize her for being different? Will it penalize her by shaping the perceptions of the adults around her, the educators and therapists and paraprofessionals who work with her, who are supposed to teach her and help her learn? My fear is that it does not provide them with information to guide how they reach her or connect with her, but rather provides them with the evidence to unwittingly justify lowering their expectations, to console themselves with assurances that they're doing all they can, to tell themselves it's pointless—the student is "below average."

Despite the appalling lack of resources invested into public schools, the increasingly large class sizes, the insufficient number of adequately trained teachers, the demoralizingly low compensation for paraprofessionals, and an array of other institutional or structural problems, the deficit, ironically, becomes located in Michaela, not in the system.

5 Belonging

The summer after Michaela turned six years old, I found myself at a playground with all three of my children. Aidric and I had ridden our bikes, and I'd pulled Michaela and Zora in our red bike trailer, battered from years of use. The trailer had been a hand-me-down, and since Aidric was about a year old, I have used it regularly, first pulling him, then pulling him and Michaela. By the time Zora was ready to sit safely in the trailer, Aidric could ride independently, so now I pulled Michaela and Zora. During the first summer of COVID-19 lockdowns, we rode to just about every playground and outdoor destination imaginable.

This day, shortly after our arrival, two other children ran up to the playground. Aidric, Michaela, and Zora were climbing the pretend rock wall and tumbling down plastic slides. Aidric soon began playing with a girl about a year older than him. He introduced himself and then his siblings. The girl had noticed Michaela. Kids about Aidric's age appear to pause and contemplate Michaela—her sometimes halting use of language, rocky pronunciation of certain words, mannerisms that don't strictly follow tacit social norms, perhaps the trademark physical features. But I've found that other children are not generally put off by it. They may observe for a moment, since kids are tremendously curious about the world they inhabit, but they don't assign special meanings to her personality or identity unless adults around them do so first. Normally, it's the parents who seem confused, and from a place of uncertainty their default reaction is avoidance. Children, by contrast, just take it in and then figure out how best to interact with Michaela. I contemplated this as I stepped off to the side to allow the kids space to play together, wanting to give them some autonomy. But I couldn't help but eavesdrop on the conversation that ensued.

"My name is Aidric," he said. "I'm seven years old. Almost eight. My birthday is in August. My talent is running and jumping." I raised an eyebrow and wondered why he was suddenly listing physical abilities.

"That girl down there is Zora, my sister," said Aidric, after he climbed to an upper level of the jungle gym. "Her talent is fighting."

I chuckled and couldn't help but agree. Zora is a spitfire and it's not unknown for her to bully Aidric, who is twice her age and twice her size. It's usually not a violent or aggressive form of fighting, not something fueled by hostility or outright meanness. She's just forceful when she wants to be. Daring. Tough. Adventurous. All good qualities.

"My other sister is Michaela," continued Aidric.

I listened intently, wondering how he would describe her.

A brief, contemplative pause.

"We haven't figured out her talent yet."

I was awestruck, and not because he couldn't think of something. Michaela does everything her siblings do. She runs, jumps, climbs, rides. She has no limits at the playground. She fights with her brother and sister and often dominates wrestling matches. Yet it is true that Michaela does not run as fast as Aidric or climb as well as Zora, who is two years younger. She tires more quickly, needs to rest more, especially on hot days. Aidric was riding a bike independently at an age when she still uses training wheels. When Zora wants to get away, Michaela struggles to catch her.

But Aidric did not focus on any of these perceived weaknesses or delays. He did not resort to listing deficiencies, to comparing her to some assumed average or norm. He simply reasoned that we haven't figured out her talents yet. It's not that she does not have talents. We have simply failed to identify them.

That summer when I sat observing my children play, Michaela already six years old, I no longer viewed her as a child with Down syndrome. I'm not sure when it happened. Like many forms of change, it was a process, a combination of purposeful reflection and just being swept up in the flow of life—settling into new routines, normalizing what had once seemed unfathomable. But within the first year or two, I stopped seeing Down syndrome every time I looked at Michaela.

At their ages, too, eight and four years old, Aidric and Zora do not view Michaela through the lens of disability. We periodically talk to them about Down syndrome and let them know they can always ask questions, preparing them with vocabulary and conceptual tools to navigate life as siblings of a sister with Down syndrome. But it's not something Aidric ever asks about. Zora is still too young for those sorts of conversations, though we've started mentioning to her that sometimes Michaela needs a little more guidance. But for Aidric and Zora, Michaela is not a sister with Down syndrome. She is just their sister. In our day-to-day family life, Michaela is not a child with Down syndrome. She is a sibling, a daughter, a friend. She is Michaela.

These moments of stunning openness and acceptance punctuate the daily drama of parenting, filled with frustrating flashes of kids fighting, pushing boundaries, and refusing to cooperate. It's both amazing and overwhelming. As Alison Piepmeier writes, describing her own experience as a mother of a daughter with Down syndrome, parenting in general is difficult, "not the specifics of parenting a child with Down syndrome."[1]

During the same summer as that park visit, Zora had an abscessed front tooth, mysteriously damaged weeks earlier, extracted. Still woozy from the procedure as we returned home, she proudly marched in the house with three bouncy balls, her prize from the dental office for being a cooperative patient. She had insisted on getting one each for Aidric and Michaela. I ushered them and their projectiles outside and grabbed my shoes, sitting on the porch to put them on. I watched all three kids bounce the balls higher and higher off the driveway. Before long, Aidric bounced one over the house and into the backyard. They all ran after it. I went through the house and came out the back to help them find the ball in the long grass and weeds. We don't even have much of a yard in back. It's mostly a wooded hillside that slopes down to a lake. As we looked around, I realized Michaela wasn't with us. I glanced down the hill to make sure she wasn't headed toward the water, then dashed back into the house and into the garage, and finally into the driveway. I spotted her down the block on a bicycle, several houses down, heading toward an intersection that marks the edge of our neighborhood. The cross street doesn't usually have heavy traffic, but with no stop signs, the periodic car sometimes drives at high speed. A curve in the street and gentle slopes in the road also make it difficult to spot a fast-approaching car. Michaela only occasionally looks for cars and often has her head facing down when she rides a bike. All my kids are prohibited from crossing past that street on their own, and one of my missions in life is to teach them to religiously stop at the intersection and look carefully for cars.

I sprinted down the street to catch up with Michaela. She was riding a pedal-less balance bike, dark red frame with small black tires, on which she is impressively fast, and wearing a white toy astronaut helmet, tinted visor pulled down. As I ran down the street at full speed, she turned into the last house's driveway before the intersection and then rode into the grass, zigzagging between a row of tall pine trees with skinny trunks. I slowed down, relieved she wasn't headed into potential danger.

"Michaela, what are you doing?" I asked, catching my breath as I strolled toward her.

"I'm looking for Zach! Where's Zach?"

"Who is Zach," I asked?

"Aidric is Zach," she responded, slightly annoyed, as if I should have known already.

"Oh, are you pretending to be the Wild Kratts," I asked?

The *Wild Kratts* is a popular PBS Kids show, featuring the real-life Kratt brothers, Martin and Chris, who teach viewers about wild animals, then narrate an animated adventure with cartoon versions of themselves competing with a rotation of villains, one of whom is named Zach Varmitech, a whiny, irritable genius who tries to dominate nature with technology. Michaela likes to pretend to be Aviva Corcovado, the bold engineer who accompanies the Kratt brothers on their adventures and invents all their creature power suits, which allow them to take on the special powers of certain animals to battle with villains such as Zach.

"Yes! Aidric is Zach!"

Interesting, I thought. Whatever might this say about her perception of her older brother?

I convinced her that Aidric/Zach was still at home, and she agreed to ride back. We had been bouncing balls, Michaela had been playing Wild Kratts. What is called "elopement" by professionals has been something of a minor challenge with Michaela in recent years. Sometimes the behavior is referred to as bolting.[2] But she doesn't take off randomly, as if she has no idea what she's doing, so that's not an accurate term. Rather, she gets an idea in her head, just wants to go for a bike ride or explore something, and then acts on the impulse. One time she ran down a bowling alley lane, straight for the triangle assortment of pins at the end. Another time, when I was waiting with her during Aidric's soccer practice at an elementary school gymnasium, she removed her clothes and ran down a hallway lined with other parents. They looked up and watched. I suddenly felt embarrassed by the sting of public shame, objectified by their gazes as Michaela transgressed behavioral norms and I rushed to restore her "proper" public behavior by chasing after her.

I have come to realize that my experience of shame reflects the ableist attitudes and practices that police our behavior in social settings. Ableism describes assumptions and attitudes that reinforce notions of normality and devalue those who fall outside its parameters. As disability studies scholar Fiona Campbell writes, we live in a world where we constantly learn "that to be disabled is to be *less than*, a world where disability may be *tolerated* but in the final instance, is *inherently negative*."[3] In such a world, a child with disabilities is "watched" and stared at in ways that other children are not. From the reproachful glance to the hard, judgmental stare, parents of children with disabilities, and disabled persons themselves, frequently confront the scrutiny of others who unwittingly and silently seek to enforce ableist norms. The stare itself sends the message: *you are out of line.* After our family attended a party at a friend's house, for instance, a colleague felt compelled to tell me how surprised they were that Michaela seemed like such a "normal" child compared to the other kids present. I had no idea they were so closely watching her.[4]

Elopement is one of those transgressive behaviors that can reveal unspoken ableist norms, the world of take-for-granted cultural expectations made obvious by my own embarrassed reactions or those of others watching. While sometimes elopement is impulsive, other times it is calculated, a way to get attention, with Michaela relishing the excitement of me chasing her down a school hallway or down the street as she approaches the intersection. I unintentionally reinforce the behavior with my frenzied reactions, chasing her, calling her back, with my own reaction of embarrassment. It makes it exciting, so she does it more. Sometimes you have no choice but to give chase for safety reasons, but if I just ignored her, such elopement would likely diminish. This behavior has been improving as she gets older and I learn to cope with the ableist gaze of others, but it's still annoying.

It's especially frustrating when Zora does it. As a fiercely independent four-year-old, she feels entitled to leave on her bike like her older brother and she takes joy in defying me. As Michaela and I walked back to the house, Zora suddenly appeared in the front yard wearing nothing but her underwear. Earlier in the day she had taken her clothes off and sat under the kitchen table drawing lines over much of her legs and arms with black pen. Now her clothes were off again. Holding Michaela's hand, I looked up to see Zora scurry through the yard and into the street. As she ran away, I also noticed she had peed a little, leaving a wet spot on her backside. Some of our neighbors, a retired couple who walk their cat around the neighborhood, watched silently as she ran past them into the street, little wet butt, inked-up body, and missing front tooth. She screeched joyfully as I chased after her. I was not laughing. The cat stared at us from the curb.

This, from my neurotypical four-year-old. Hilarious in retrospect, exasperating in the moment.

.   .   .   .   .

Parenting, of course, is filled with such experiences, situations that puzzle and frustrate, that compel us to discover new wellsprings of patience and understanding. I bet this is a truism for all parents, regardless of their child's chromosomes. When I think about the family of Erik Erikson, I can only wonder what Neil's talents were, if he ever played at a neighborhood park, dashed off on a bike, or sprinted through the yard in his underwear, if he ever had a chance to push boundaries and test social norms, if he ever frustrated caretakers with creative, joyful imagination. His story will likely never be known.

We do know that the decision to institutionalize Neil in 1944 was deeply corrosive for the Erikson family, a trauma with lifelong impact. It fed distrust and anguish. After telling their three other children that Neil had died at birth, Erik and Joan avoided discussion of what happened. No attempt to mourn the unexpected loss, no rituals of grieving to help cope with death. It was a loss that never happened, a life nonexistent.

Joan had been shut out of the decision to send Neil away, which occurred while she was unconscious, a terribly misplaced effort to protect her from the presumed pain of bonding with a flawed newborn whom doctors assumed she would surely lose anyway. She was devastated by this decision. Joan later questioned Erik, challenging the necessity of keeping Neil away. She insisted on visiting him.[5] During the first year, Joan had Neil transferred between a few different private caretakers, before admitting him to a public institution in California. His existence was rarely acknowledged beyond that, revealed to only a few close friends. Neil was never photographed, his features undocumented. In his absence, the Eriksons portrayed their family life to the outside world as idyllic, "a healthy, attractive, and vibrant family headed by a young child analyst," as recounted by Erikson's biographer.[6] They maintained a beautiful suburban home in the foothills of California, swimming pool and gardens, frequently hosting guests. Behind closed doors, the relationship between Erik and Joan became fragmented and filled with sorrow, strained by emotional distance.[7] The pain of losing a child, but especially the guilt of abandoning him, would torment Joan for life.[8]

With their other children, Erik and Joan maintained a pattern of silence around Neil for years. When Neil was seven, his siblings now teenagers, they finally told all of them, amid moving the family from California back to the East Coast. Erik Erikson had recently published his first famous book, *Childhood and Society,* making him an intellectual celebrity, and he accepted first a new position at the Austen Riggs Center in Massachusetts, then one at Harvard. The decision to move away, with Neil remaining in a California institution, was partly an attempt to distance themselves from the trauma of his existence.[9] For youngest siblings Jon and Sue, they were leaving their mysterious brother behind. Their parents discouraged them from trying to visit Neil, describing him as "terribly deformed."[10] Even after Erik and Joan revealed the truth of Neil's existence, the family never talked about him.

In her memoir titled *In the Shadow of Fame,* Sue recalls feeling a profound sense of unreconciled loss when she believed that Neil had died, and that loss transforming into a fear of abandonment when she learned the truth. The sense of loss emanated from the transformed relationship with her mother. As a five-year-old child, Sue had bonded with her pregnant mother over the pending arrival of Neil, a bond that dissolved when his birth did not occur as expected.

"I had lost the baby that she and I were to care for together," writes Sue, "and I had lost the opportunity to bond with her in this special way. But worst of all, my mother had withdrawn from me into her own terrible pain. I was on my own with mine."[11]

When Sue was thirteen, Joan divulged that Neil was still alive as they were driving through the endless desert landscape of New Mexico, a desolate stretch of the long trip eastward. "We were leaving Neil behind," Sue writes, "emotionally as well as geographically."[12] Sue recalls struggling to trust her parents, feeling as though she too might become a source of shame, perhaps left behind somewhere. The specter of emotional exile haunted her relationship with her parents.

"The memory of Neil's exile hung always over my careful relationship with Mom and Dad," writes Sue. "Neil's birth and existence had caused them such shame and guilt that they banished him from awareness. I, too, experienced their pained withdrawal when something I said or did threatened their fragile sense of themselves. On some level I always feared the possibility of excommunication."[13]

Neil died in 1965, a young man. Erik and Joan were in Italy when they found out, taking a call while hosting a dinner with close friends who already knew of Neil. They briefly mentioned the matter then resumed the dinner as if nothing extraordinary happened. Neil's remains were to be cremated, and they asked Sue and Jon to arrange for the burial of his ashes. They did not return from Italy for the funeral, their son ignored in death as in life.[14]

"Jon and I selected a cemetery we thought attractive in a nearby town," recalls Sue. "And as we discussed the burial arrangement with the cemetery staff, we were embarrassed to reveal that we knew nothing about the brother we were laying to rest."[15]

They asked that Neil be buried in the children's section of the cemetery. The eternal child. His identity to them was an ableist stereotype forged through society's changing understanding of Down syndrome.

"We watched as Neil's urn was placed in the ground," Sue recounts, "feeling this must surely be a dream. We spoke to him and to each other of our sadness that he had been excluded from our family life, acknowledging that we could not be sure we would have wanted him to come live with us back in 1944, even if we had known that he was alive. How could we know that? But we were sure about the ongoing guilt and sorrow we felt toward the brother we had never been permitted to know or to love."[16]

.   .   .   .   .

In some ways, the world Neil left was very different from the one he had entered. In the 1930s, the British scientist Lionel Penrose had already begun publishing statistical analyses questioning the hereditary and racialized assumptions associated with mongolism, pointing instead to maternal age as a risk factor and theorizing a "chromosome aberration" as a potential explanation.[17] Over the 1950s and 1960s, the development of clinical genetics enabled new techniques for visualizing the structure of the human chromosome. The discovery of new solutions to prepare microscope slide samples allowed for clearly seeing that the diploid number of chromosomes in humans is typically forty-six. It was then in 1959 that French scientists Jérôme LeJeune and Marthe Gautier found the trisomy of the twenty-first chromosome in people still classified as mongoloid. Two years later, *The Lancet* published a letter signed by nineteen prominent doctors who called for abandoning the terms mongolism, mongoloid, or Mongolian idiocy.[18] The intent was to escape the pejorative racial connotations and other stigma associated with earlier terminology. Within the English-speaking world, the term Down syndrome was slowly adopted over the next couple of decades. As it became increasingly understood as a genetic condition, the racial undertones previously emphasized by the eugenics movement diminished. Neil Erikson was born with mongolism but died with Down syndrome.

The understanding of Down syndrome as a genetic condition unfolded alongside advances in reproductive technologies in the 1960s and 1970s, particularly the ability to prenatally screen a fetus for potential chromosomal conditions through technologies such as amniocentesis and chorionic villus sampling (CVS). By the late 1940s, medical doctors knew that they could determine a fetus's sex by examining the fetal cells found in fluid drawn from a pregnant person's amniotic sac. In 1966, researchers conducted the first karyotyping of fetal cells obtained through amniocentesis, opening the door to the procedure's use in prenatal testing for conditions such as Down syndrome.[19] CVS, which involves a biopsy of the placenta for genetic analysis, was also developed in the 1970s, becoming widely available by the 1980s.

Just as parents were pushing for inclusion of their disabled children in the community and as the normalization movement began to transform conventional thinking around intellectual and cognitive disability, new prenatal screening technologies began to target conditions such as Down syndrome, justified through a mixture of eugenic and economic arguments. The dominant medical paradigm of the era saw prenatal screening as a tool to help identify and eliminate fetuses with "defects," reducing the supposed future burden on society by reducing the number of people destined for institutionalization.[20] Even though Down syndrome was now being understood as a random genetic condition, emerging medical discourses still framed it as a deeply undesirable abnormality, and one that could be eliminated by new biomedical technologies.

In 1968, for instance, the *Atlantic Monthly* published a heartwrenching story by Bernard Bard, a reporter for the *New York Post* and a father whose son, like Michaela, was diagnosed with Down syndrome days after birth. Bard describes the trauma and sense of loss he felt as the diagnosis sunk in, an experience all too familiar to me. Doctors encouraged him and his wife to institutionalize their child, whom they had named Philip. No treatment or cure could help their Philip, he was told, and if their son even lived beyond a few years, caring for him would be unfair to their "normal" children. If Philip happened to live into adulthood, he would burden their family for a lifetime. Medical research, doctors said, was focusing on how to "eliminate the prenatal causes of mongolism." Bard then recounts arranging for his son to be sent to a private institution. When he visited, he found children languishing in dark, dreary rooms. Nurses told him Philip would receive daily care, but nothing to "artifi-

cially" prolong his life, no inoculations against childhood diseases, no surgeries, not even basic medical interventions like oxygen for respiratory
issues. Not long after a social worker transferred Philip to the institution,
the managing doctor called to inform Bard that his son had died from
"heart failure and jaundice."

"Consider it a blessing," he recounted the doctor saying.

In telling his story, Bard conveys emotional conflict, a father struggling
to cope with complex feelings of guilt and the shame of abandoning his
son, including the confusion of his mysterious death, but he does not
attribute Philip's demise to institutional neglect. The entire narrative
frames parents like Bard as the victims of a preventable fate, suggesting
their suffering could be diminished if children with Down syndrome were
never born. He calls for a humane approach to euthanasia. "I do not know
how it should be practiced," he concludes, "or what committee should have
a voice in the decisions, or what pill or injection might best be employed.
I do know that there are thousands of children on this earth who should
never have been born. Their lives are a blank. They do not play; they do
not read; they do not grow; they do not live or love. Their life is without
meaning to themselves, and an agony to their families. Why?"[21]

*Their lives are a blank. They do not play; they do not read; they do not
grow; they do not live or love. Michaela does all these things, and lives with
richness others long for.*

Bard's story was followed in the *Atlantic Monthly* article by a response
from Joseph Fletcher, who at the time was a prominent theologian and
professor at the Episcopal Theological School in Cambridge,
Massachusetts. He elaborates an argument in support of Bard, suggesting
we should not "quit in dumb resignation to that mysterious, disastrous
forty-seventh chromosome." He celebrates how the institution in Bard's
account did nothing to "keep death away. On the contrary, it is welcomed
as a friend." Fletcher acknowledges and, incredibly, endorses the implied
neglect as "indirect euthanasia." "In dealing with Down's cases," writes
Fletcher, "it is obvious that the end everybody wants is death." He also
addresses the deep sorrow that Bard conveyed in his story about Philip.
"People in Bard's situation," Fletcher continues, "have no reason to feel
guilty about putting a Down's syndrome baby away, whether it's 'put away'
in the sense of hidden in a sanitarium or in a more responsible lethal

sense. It is sad; yes. Dreadful. But it carries no guilt. True guilt arises only from an offense against a person, and a Down's is not a person."[22]

It is tough for me to read that last line, a naked statement of callous beliefs condoning infanticide, asserted as some sort of scientific fact or as universally accepted common sense. *Not a person.* It grates against my lived reality today. Michaela's personhood was perhaps in doubt in the confusing moments after her diagnosis, but I always knew we would bring her home and care for her. The doubt faded. She quickly became a loving part of our family. She is creative, imaginative, caring.

We don't know all her talents yet, but we will.

As extreme as Fletcher's ideas might sound these days, in 1968 the *Atlantic Monthly* article elicited little backlash and Fletcher would later become a professor of medical ethics at the University of Virginia School of Medicine. His views were in line with medical practices at the time. Withholding basic medical care to babies with Down syndrome was routine, particularly as pediatric medicine improved. By the 1960s, pediatric cardiology was widespread in the United States.[23] Once life-threatening issues such as congenital heart defects, which occur in about half of all babies born with Down syndrome, could be corrected with surgery. But many doctors and even parents found it logical to withhold lifesaving medical treatments from such babies, leaving them to die.[24] Others viewed such surgeries as training for the real thing. The 1970 memoir *The Making of a Surgeon*, by William Nolen, recounts a conversation between a pediatrician and a young surgeon who is preparing to conduct open heart surgery the next day. The surgeon says he's not concerned about the patient dying during the procedure. "Oh, now I get it," replies the pediatrician, "you're doing a mongoloid."[25]

While stories such as Bard's continued to occur, in 1971 what became known as the "Hopkins Mongol Case" signaled a turning point in the development of modern medical ethics. In the spring of that year, a baby with Down syndrome was born at Johns Hopkins Hospital and diagnosed with duodenal atresia, an easily corrected intestinal blockage that stops food or fluid from leaving a baby's stomach. The parents refused to consent to surgery and the baby died of dehydration two weeks later, one of several deaths at Johns Hopkins involving infants with Down syndrome who had treatable conditions. Several nurses and physicians were uncomfortable with what happened, but many others in the medical profession supported the parents' decision and condoned the withholding of treatment.[26] A chief pediatrician at Johns Hopkins, Dr. Robert E. Cooke, had two daughters with cri du chat syndrome, a chromosomal condition linked to intellectual disabilities, and was personally involved in advocating for children with disabilities. Cooke was also connected to the Kennedy family, having served as a senior medical adviser to President John F. Kennedy and as family pediatrician to Eunice Kennedy Shriver. Shortly after the death of the infant with duodenal atresia, Cooke met with Shriver and the Kennedy Foundation to propose making a movie about the case. *Who Shall Survive? One of the Choices on Our Conscience* premiered in October 1971 at the newly opened Kennedy Center in Washington, DC. Dramatizing the experiences of the medical professionals involved, it began with a doctor recounting the moment the baby died, saying that "he looked very much like a child you would have found abandoned somewhere and left to die, in a garbage can." The film generated national media attention and spurred numerous publications that helped establish the emerging field of bioethics.

Yet even as new discussions about the ethics of treating children with Down syndrome unfolded in relation to the medical profession, courts continued to uphold the rights of parents to withhold treatment from their disabled children. In 1978, the California Supreme Court ruled that the parents of Philip Becker, an eleven-year-old with Down syndrome, could refuse heart surgery to repair a ventricular sepal defect. The case was peculiar because Becker had never lived at home with his parents and was under the full-time care of a foster home. In court hearings, the parents, doctors, and other experts testified about whether they thought it was worth conducting surgery to extend the life of someone with disabilities. In his ruling in favor of the parents' right to withhold treatment from their child, the judge characterized the heart surgery as "elective" and questioned the value of a life with Down syndrome.[27] Following this decision, the foster home caring for Philip sued his parents and claimed legal guardianship, which was eventually granted, and the surgery was performed.

Such controversies extended into the 1980s, with many doctors continuing to advise or support parents in refusing to consent to life-saving medical treatment of children with Down syndrome.[28] With the medical profession divided on the ethics of such situations, an infant who came to be known as Baby Doe was born on April 9, 1982, in Bloomington, Indiana. In addition to Down syndrome, Baby Doe was also born with esophageal atresia, a condition in which parts of the esophagus do not develop properly, risking that food could be inhaled into the lungs. The obstetrician who delivered Baby Doe discouraged the parents from consenting to surgery, in disagreement with the family's physician and a local pediatrician who wanted to correct the treatable condition. The physicians supporting surgery attempted legal action under state child negligence laws and recruited families willing to adopt the child, but local courts deferred to the parent's decision. While litigation progressed, Baby Doe died of dehydration and pneumonia at six days old.[29]

In response to this incident and others that came to be known as "Baby Doe cases," President Ronald Reagan's administration pushed for rules in the mid-1980s that required healthcare providers to report discrimination based on disability in decision-making about medical treatment plans. While some in the medical profession welcomed such rules, others worried that blanket federal mandates would stifle the ability of physicians and parents to make difficult decisions in cases where infants were born with extreme medical conditions considered "incompatible with life," leading to aggressive overtreatment. In 1992, for instance, in what became known as the Baby K case, a mother insisted that her infant, born with anencephaly and missing most of her brain and a portion of her skull, receive life-sustaining treatment against the advice of her doctors, who determined that such care was futile. Most infants born with anencephaly only live a few days, but based on federal Baby Doe regulations, a court ordered a hospital in Fairfax, Virginia, to provide medical treatment. Lacking cognitive function and unable to hear or see, the child lived in a pediatric nursing facility and was rushed to the emergency room to receive mechanical ventilation whenever she had trouble breathing. She died of cardiac arrest in 1995, at two years old, and the case triggered public debate over how to care for such children and who gets to decide.

When it comes down to it, no institutional rule will cover every ethically fraught scenario. The fact is, some parents do face agonizing situations in which they must decide whether and how to pursue life-sustaining treatment for terminally ill children.[30] But Down syndrome is not an illness, and that extra chromosome is certainly not a death sentence. In recent decades, healthcare professional bodies have sought to strike a balance, embracing the ethical standard that disability should not be a justification for withholding life-sustaining treatment, while also maintaining that treatment decisions should be based on the best interests of the child.[31] Down syndrome marked a turning point in these charged ethical debates, centered on how we define personhood and what it means to live a good life.

.   .   .   .   .

Even as some doctors in the late 1960s and 1970s still advised parents to institutionalize their babies with Down syndrome or encouraged them to deny medical treatment, the broader disability rights movement began to achieve important policy gains. Institutionalization was coming under persistent critique, and new programs were taking shape to help parents raise their children with Down syndrome at home and then support them in school. Public attitudes were changing and the growing visibility of children with Down syndrome in popular culture further humanized the condition.

Like others who had shared their stories through personal memoirs in order to challenge dominant beliefs and assert the personhood of their children with disabilities, parent advocates such as Emily Perl Kingsley helped change how a new generation would view intellectual disability.[32] In 1974, Kingsley gave birth to her son Jason, who was soon diagnosed with Down syndrome. Doctors offered a gloomy prognosis still typical for the era and advised institutionalization, suggesting she and her husband tell others their baby had died during childbirth. They brought Jason home instead. After a few weeks, Kingsley came across an advertisement in a newspaper for a local group for parents of children with Down syndrome. She and her husband attended, and they discovered people full of enthusiasm and eager to share their experiences. They found connection and friendship, families celebrating their children with Down syndrome, families embracing difference.

When Jason was born, Kingsley had already been a writer for the new children's educational show *Sesame Street*, starting in 1970, a year after it first aired. *Sesame Street* was an innovative experiment at the time, aimed at preschool children and informed by research on early childhood education. The creators had already been having discussions about how to include children with disabilities and Jason first appeared on the show when he was fifteen months old. "At first," writes cocreator Joan Ganz Cooney, "we also did separate segments with curriculum and activities for children with special learning needs. But we learned quickly that these children didn't need a different format. So our next step was to demonstrate that they did not need to be segregated in special education programs but could be part of a regular elementary school class."[33]

Over the years, Jason made several appearances on *Sesame Street*, along with other children with Down syndrome. He was also featured in an hour-long NBC special in 1977 called *This Is My Son*, as well as an award-winning made-for-TV movie that premiered on CBS in 1987 called *Kids like These*, written by Kingsley. These sorts of initiatives marked a significant turning point, propelling Down syndrome into mass media and popular visual culture. Children with Down syndrome were no longer in the shadows. In 1994, Jason Kingsley would publish *Count Us In: Growing Up with Down Syndrome*, co-authored with Mitchell Levitz. People with Down syndrome were speaking for themselves.

Parents such as Emily Perl Kingsley were no longer writing memoirs about the dilemma of institutionalization, as an earlier generation of parents had, but telling stories about the challenges of inclusion and the realization of new policy reforms that guaranteed access to schools. They were contributing to a cultural revolution that asserted the personhood of their children with Down syndrome, emphasizing belonging, not difference, imagining and building a new world entirely. As recounted in the book *Life as We Know It: A Father, a Family, and an Exceptional Child*, when Michael Bérubé and Janet Lyon's second child Jamie was born with Down syndrome in 1991, it came as a surprise and Jamie needed emergency medical treatment. "We can handle this," Janet said.[34]

By the 1990s, at the start of the post-ADA generation, popular culture was increasingly representing Down syndrome in positive terms. Children with Down syndrome were routinely attending neighborhood schools and visible within the community. The parent groups that had organized decades earlier had laid the groundwork for the establishment of local support groups in many communities across the United States. Organizations like The Arc and the Down Syndrome Association of Wisconsin, among others, nurture local groups and cultivate informal parent-to-parent networking. Such networks supply not only information and practical resources, but also emotional support, helping new parents to cope with altered expectations or the ableist attitudes that continue to stigmatize children with disabilities. "Collectively through their activism," writes anthropologist Rayna Rapp, "parents of children with Down syndrome developed, deployed, and transmitted a worldview in which difference could be accepted and a new identity as parents of a different child could be formulated and assumed."[35] This is also a process of constructing a new form of community around Down syndrome, parents finding support then friendship with others who share similar life experiences.

Bérubé, a literary scholar, would write about the experience of Jamie's birth and first few years for *Harper's Magazine* in 1994, and then in his 1996 book *Life as We Know It*. Part memoir, part social commentary, books like this helped to establish new terms for discussion, framing Down syndrome not as a chromosomal defect or medical illness, but as a form of genetic variation, human biology intersecting with cultural ideologies that define who belongs and who doesn't. Other such books would follow, marking a new genre of memoir that challenges the very terms of belonging and cultivates alternative visions of the future.[36]

Such books are both intellectual and therapeutic. I began to discover them in the weeks and months after Michaela's birth, reading them to get some perspective on my experience, to come to terms with the sense of disorientation, to rethink my own assumptions about our life ahead. These books convey a worldview in which Down syndrome and disability fit among other forms of diversity, the forms of difference that have served as bases for claiming rights and asserting personhood. They constitute a toolkit for world-building.

In this world, elopement is not transgression, Down syndrome is not watched. It is welcomed.

·   ·   ·   ·   ·

"In dealing with Down's cases, it is obvious that the end everybody wants is death."

When Fletcher wrote that line in 1968, a time when Down syndrome was gaining in public visibility and acceptance, the ethical terrain for determining whether a life with Down syndrome is a life worth living was shifting inward, from the nervous discussions between doctors and new parents to the private realm of individual choice. Amid this shift, the philosophical argument that a life with Down syndrome is not a life worth living has persisted as well, advanced by other prominent bioethicists, most notably Peter Singer, who has made claims about the supposed diminished personhood of people with Down syndrome to justify positions on infanticide and euthanasia.[37] In 1994, he wrote that "to have a child with Down syndrome is to have a very different experience from having a normal child. It can still be a warm and loving experience, but we must have lowered expectations for our child's ability."[38] In this framework, "ability" is the assumed criterion for being human, with cognitive capacity the basis for defining personhood and rights. Those "lacking," in this estimation, fail to reach the threshold of being fully human. They have less value. Their nonexistence is desirable, their elimination justifiable.[39]

The ableist fantasy of nonexistence has seemed technologically achievable in recent decades. Over the 1980s and 1990s, prenatal screening technologies such as amniocentesis were increasingly offered to pregnant people, particularly those in their late thirties, considered at higher risk for having a baby with Down syndrome. Prenatal screening marked a new intersection of technology and reproduction, with genetic knowledge becoming a basis from which to imagine pregnancy and assert control over its outcomes. In some ways, new reproductive technologies, coupled with the right to abortion, empowered women to exercise greater control and choice over their pregnancies. If prenatal screening could diagnose potential "abnormalities" of a fetus, then women could elect to end the pregnancy. But it also thrust individual women to the center of morally fraught dilemmas around how to define normality and human worth.

In 1984, the anthropologist Rayna Rapp wrote poignantly about her experience with amniocentesis for *Ms.* magazine, a publication launched a decade earlier to give voice to the women's movement. Whereas Margaret Mead had embodied a trailblazing woman who challenged conventions of gender and sexuality through her life and career, Rapp helped to establish feminist anthropology as a vibrant subfield that engaged directly with second wave feminism in the 1970s, editing the landmark volume *Toward an Anthropology of Women* in 1975. At that time, Mead was still writing for *Redbook*, which had come under critique for reinforcing conservative ideas about femininity and motherhood. *Ms.* was a militant alternative that spoke to the changing realities of women's lives.

In her essay "The Ethics of Choice," Rapp recounts the joy and excitement she and her husband experienced when she became pregnant at age thirty-six, and then the emotional devastation when she learned her fetus likely had an extra copy of the twenty-first chromosome. "Fear of Down syndrome," she writes, had motivated her to choose amniocentesis to screen for chromosomal conditions.[40] In the early 1980s, over twenty thousand women each year were electing to have the prenatal test to diagnosis conditions such as Down syndrome, Tay-Sachs disease, and sickle-cell anemia. For 98 percent of those women, the test revealed no anomalies. But Rapp's fetus was diagnosed with Down syndrome, news delivered over the phone nearly two weeks after the procedure, a long and stressful waiting period. "I began to scream as soon as I recognized her voice," writes Rapp of her doctor's call. "The image of myself, alone, screaming into a white plastic telephone is indelible." When she replays the moment in her mind, "time is suspended," her "screams echo for indefinite periods." She and her husband felt devastated. "Our fantasies for XYLO," as they had tentatively named their five-month-old fetus, "were completely shattered."[41]

I know that feeling. A phone call. Michaela's pediatrician. Erikson to Mead. Rapp's doctor. The echo, the psychological fragmentation, the distressing sense of demise, of being emotionally adrift. I have felt the weight of replaying the moment of the diagnosis repeatedly. Grief accompanies the shattering of expectations you didn't realize you had, leaving only confusion about what you lost, and uncertainty about what to do next. It is a fragile moment, lives abruptly set on new trajectories.

Before undertaking amniocentesis, Rapp and her husband had already decided they would abort a fetus with Down syndrome. Rapp was strikingly honest about the fears that motivated her decision, concerns that reflect the dominant attitudes of the 1980s. She feared Down syndrome would entail a lifetime of "burdens" for her and "likely" suffering for her child, whom she assumed would rely on modern medical technologies to "keep them alive." She worried about the challenges of "raising a child who could never grow to independence" and having to "transform" herself to become a full-time advocate in a "society where the state provides virtually no decent, humane services" for people with intellectual disabilities. "Most women who've opted for amniocentesis," writes Rapp, "are prepared to face the question of abortion, and many of us *do* choose it, after diagnosis of serious disability is made. Perhaps 95 percent of Down syndrome pregnancies are terminated after test results are known."[42]

Rapp values the ability to make these choices, to gather information prenatally, to abort if something has gone awry. She supports the empowerment of women to control their bodies and reproductive lives. But she also acknowledges the stunning, life-altering impact of exercising these rights and how new reproductive technologies had placed her at the crossroads of an altogether new phenomenon: Women like her were among the first generation to come of age with amniocentesis, plunged into a lonely ethical morass of having to determine what types of "lives are worth living."[43] This compounded the emotional trauma of losing an otherwise desired fetus. "I had no idea that deep mourning for a fetus could be so disorienting." She found that "to end the life of a fetus you've wanted and carried for most of five months" was followed by enormous psychological pain.[44] This is an ordeal that many women endure alone. Knowing this, Rapp offered her story in a spirit of feminist solidarity, the creation of shared experience and understanding for a generation of women on the front lines of making such choices.

The trauma that Rapp experienced became the basis for a research project that examined the social impact and cultural meanings of amniocentesis. Following her experience, over the next decade she interviewed hundreds of women, observed genetic counselors advising patients about amniocentesis, probed why some women did or did not elect for prenatal screening, and why many ended a pregnancy after a positive diagnosis. The resulting book, *Testing Women, Testing the Fetus: The Social Impact of Amniocentesis in America*, documented how amniocentesis became increasingly routine over the 1980s and 1990s, but continued to obligate women to engage in difficult ethical decision-making, enrolling them as private judges of normality, placing them one by one at "the intersection of personal pain and national political struggles concerning health care, abortion rights, and disability rights."[45]

Amniocentesis unfolded in a context where individuals and institutions—mothers and families—still experienced pressures to "produce normatively acceptable babies," babies who embody cultural ideals about success, achievement, and progress.[46] As prenatal screening became routine, it was accompanied by sterile medical language and a parched logic of risk management, embodied by a new category of medical professionals known as genetic counselors. In contrast to earlier decades, by the 1990s doctors no longer approached Down syndrome as a condition that necessitated immediately removing a baby from its mother, as in Neil Erikson's time. Society was more inclusive, accommodating. Prenatal genetic testing, it was asserted, does not produce judgment, only information, facts delivered by seemingly neutral doctors and impartial genetic counselors. But the language of risk often does the work of casting judgement, even if that is not the conscious intent. Prenatal genetic testing seeks knowledge about "abnormalities" and "defects," knowledge concerning the presence of an extra chromosome presented as a statistic, as a probability of physical health problems or intellectual disabilities, as determinative of a future, a "defective" existence. In medical risk parlance, Down syndrome is "compatible with life," but "compatible" marks a reality apart from "ideal," a step away from "desirable."[47] The medical language of risk creates distance and separation, turning difference into pathology.

Rapp refers to the women who grapple with having to decide which types of lives are worth living as "moral pioneers." Selective abortion, she argues, "is ethically different from abortion in general." She continues, writing that although "we might want to argue that the fraught, contradictory, and technological spectacle of current abortion politics in the United States turns all aborters into moral philosophers, abortion after positive diagnosis [of Down syndrome] carries specific ethical charges. Ending a pregnancy to which one is already committed because of a particular diagnosed disability forces each woman to act as a moral philosopher of the limits, adjudicating the standards guarding entry into the human community for which she serves as normalizing gatekeeper."[48] With technologies like amniocentesis, the pursuit of normalcy became individualized, no longer the target of collective eugenics campaigns or state policy, no longer the goal of institutionalized neglect or denial of medical treatment, but the outcome of personal choices, an individual woman deciding what's best for herself or her family, deciding whether an extra chromosome is abnormal or merely inconsequential.

. . .

Around 2001, the hundredth anniversary of Margaret Mead's birth, I attended a conference at Barnard College in honor of Mead's legacy, and heard Rapp speak in person. I was a twenty-three-year-old graduate student in Binghamton, New York, visiting New York City for the first time, feeling intimidated and out of place at the prestigious Columbia University. Many students were in attendance, dressed in the urban hipster styles of the early 2000s: old leather shoes, dark yet faded skinny jeans, tweed jackets, and scarves around their necks. I was wearing blue jeans and a sweatshirt, along with sneakers. "We're painted," my friend said, noting the obvious—we did not fit in.

I was still trying to find my place in anthropology as well as life, years away from parenthood, and I found myself in a packed hall listening to Rapp give a presentation about the legacy of Mead and its relationship to the rise of feminist anthropology in the 1970s and 1980s. Mead was sometimes slow to align herself with the goals and tactics of the women's movement in the 1970s, and her evolving views expressed in *Redbook* often came across as old-fashioned. But in other ways Mead was ahead of her time and anticipated issues that would come to preoccupy feminist anthropology and the broader field in the 1990s and 2000s, and Mead had a public relevance, including access to publishing and media platforms, that many anthropologists long for.

Rapp spoke quickly and with intense intelligence, a sense of purpose that I found inspiring, emphasizing that Mead's legacy informs contemporary feminist anthropology, including her own research over the years. "Mead's insistence on the plasticity of the life cycle and the cultural context within which sexuality, marriage and reproduction are structured," explained Rapp, "and, in turn, structure individual and group experiences, was the foundation on which much of early feminist anthropology was built."[49] Mead's legacy was also "transformed in the work of feminist scholars on reproduction," such as Rapp's own analysis of new reproductive technologies.[50] Through her life experiences and research, Rapp had come to occupy an unexpected intersection between anthropology and disability consciousness.

The connections she was drawing between Mead and the work of contemporary feminist anthropologists didn't really register with me. The significance of amniocentesis and the fraught ethical choices described by Rapp similarly felt distant and impersonal. I didn't yet understand what this all meant—couldn't, really. I was too much of an outsider and lacked the pounding lived experience through which such insight makes sense. I see now, some twenty years later, how Mead's relationship to early disability rights activism, established through her engagement with parent advocacy movements in the 1950s and 1960s, and her evolving understanding of disability as a human experience worthy of anthropological attention in and of itself, anticipated the overlap of anthropology and disability studies embodied by Rapp's own life and research.[51] It also anticipated a still-unresolved predicament: Do prenatal screening technologies such as amniocentesis, asked Rapp in 1984, and support for abortion rights as a central feminist issue, "conflict with our commitment to build a better world for disabled people?"[52]

．　　．　　．　　．　　．

I first read Rapp's book *Testing Women, Testing the Fetus* as a young graduate student, roughly the same period when I heard her speak at Barnard College, a point in my life in which I was not yet attuned to the true significance of what she described, to screams that echo into an indefinite future. The phone call would come later. When I first read it, I noticed that she had dedicated the book to the memory of XYLO. I interpreted her choice to abort as common sense and the dedication as touching.

Many years later, a few weeks after Michaela was born, I sat in a restaurant with Tiffani, waiting for our lunch to arrive. Michaela's diagnosis had placed me at my own intersection of anthropology and disability consciousness, and I still felt as if I had been run over by a bus. Aidric was at daycare and the sun was shining through large windows next to our booth.

Even though we had just had our second child, Tiffani's body still recovering from months of transformation and the wounds of childbirth, family members had already asked us, gently, indirectly, if we would be trying for another. Maybe they were not conscious of this, perhaps it was not their explicit intent, but I couldn't help but feel as if we were being asked whether we would try one more time for a "normal" baby. Even our pediatrician had brought up the question of more children, to note that having a baby with Down syndrome increased our risk that future pregnancies would also have a similar outcome.

"You have about a one in a one hundred chance of having another baby with Down syndrome," I recall her stating flatly. "If you decide to get pregnant again, you'll want to pursue genetic counseling first."

Our conversation wandered. We chatted about Aidric's daycare and whether he seemed to like his teacher. We spoke about office politics in my department on campus. We spoke about our parents and the different ways they had reacted, or not, to the news of Michaela's diagnosis of Down syndrome a month earlier. We spoke of the Birth-to-3 program she had recently been enrolled in. We spoke of a life ahead. At some point, one of us commented on our pediatrician's remark about genetic counseling prior to future pregnancies.

"Well," I said, "if you ever got pregnant again, we'd have to go for genetic counseling."

"What does that entail?" asked Tiffani.

I didn't know for sure but thought of Rayna Rapp's book and the decision she had made to abort her pregnancy after a prenatal diagnosis of Down syndrome.

When Tiffani had been pregnant with Aidric a few years prior, she had selected an obstetrician available through the hospital network covered by her employer health insurance at the time. Her doctor was incredibly skilled at obstetrics, and when the time came to deliver Aidric, she had coached Tiffani through childbirth with unexpected passion and empathy. But as an obstetrician, she was also steeped in a model of childbirth that emphasizes frequent medical intervention and management, an experience Tiffani found alienating. When she later became pregnant with Michaela, she opted for a family practice doctor. He seemed a compromise, less invested in the numerous medical interventions increasingly typical of obstetrics, but still a medical doctor who delivered at the local hospital birthing center, which Tiffani preferred. She was considered "low risk" for something like Down syndrome and never pursued prenatal screening for chromosomal conditions. During ultrasounds, as with each pregnancy, we asked not to be informed about the fetus's genitalia. We didn't want to emphasize something like that, a feature that doesn't matter to us.

"If you got pregnant again," I suggested to Tiffani as I took a bite out of my salmon sandwich glazed with teriyaki sauce, "you'd have to undergo prenatal screening."

"Why is that?"

"Because of the risk of Down syndrome," I said matter-of-factly. "We'd have to know so that we could end the pregnancy."

"We?"

I looked up from my food. She was not eating.

"Um, yeah."

Her eyes swelled with tears.

"So, you're saying you don't think Michaela should have been born?"

I don't recall what I said at this point. I knew Tiffani was supportive of abortion rights in principle, including the right of women to end pregnancies after prenatal testing. And I assumed it was the obvious thing to do in cases of Down syndrome. I hadn't yet made the connection to my own daughter, asleep in her infant carrier as we spoke.

Cases of Down syndrome.

Tiffani would tell me a few years later that this was one of the lowest points in our relationship, a point at which she questioned whether she really knew me anymore. And I had begun to question whether I knew myself.

·   ·   ·   ·   ·

Even though we never sought prenatal testing when Tiffani was pregnant with Michaela, if we had done so, the test itself would have been easier than ever. When Rayna Rapp underwent amniocentesis in the 1980s, she endured a long and intense process. Her prenatal testing occurred between the sixteenth and twentieth week of pregnancy, entailed a needle being inserted though her abdomen to withdraw amniotic fluid, and carried a small risk of miscarriage. After waiting two more weeks until she received results, Rapp then underwent a second-trimester abortion, an emotionally arduous loss in which her previously visible and desired pregnancy was ended.

By the time Tiffani was pregnant with Michaela, additional screening technologies had hit the market, often known as noninvasive prenatal testing or screening (NIPT or NIPS). Based on a simple blood test, NIPT looks at pieces of placental DNA that circulate in the mother's blood. It entails a routine blood draw from the mother after nine weeks of pregnancy and results may arrive in a few days. NIPT can be done relatively early in pregnancy, is quick and easy, and is advertised as highly accurate, especially for conditions such as trisomy 21. Collecting a blood sample from the mother poses no risk to the fetus—except if it has Down syndrome.

Biotech companies have invested heavily in NIPT. Companies that sell NIPT argue that the prenatal blood test is not meant to be diagnostic, but only to identify high-risk patients in need of additional testing, such as amniocentesis or CVS. After a NIPT result suggesting high risk, such diagnostic follow-up testing should come next, but doesn't always happen. Amniocentesis and CVS can't occur until later in the pregnancy, when abortion access is more uncertain or restricted.[53]

NIPT represents a paradigm shift, a wave of new biotechnologies and forms of genetic knowledge altering how people think of themselves and others. The fantasy of knowing and controlling our genetic futures is often tethered to a narrative of "progress," one in which medical science ushers in a "better world" with more control over health and wellbeing, a promise to "improve" and "enhance." But often, explains George Estreich, a writer and father of a daughter with Down syndrome, "that narrative frames disability as a cost," something to be eliminated or edited out of existence.[54] None other than James Watson, the pioneering molecular biologist who helped discover the structure of DNA in 1953 and who was among those who developed the Human Genome Project in the early 1990s, has given voice to the fantasy of genetic perfection, achieved through elimination of those considered burdensome or unfit. "We already accept that most couples don't want a Down child," he said as part of a 2007 interview littered with racist and sexist remarks. "You would have to be crazy to say you wanted one, because that child has no future."[55]

The start of the Human Genome Project in the 1990s intensified interest in genetic information and spurred numerous enterprises geared toward not only understanding but also potentially manipulating the genes of living organisms. The CRISPR-Cas9 system, for instance, has emerged as one tool for guiding permanent changes to the DNA of living cells.[56] The development of such technologies is driven by a troubling mixture of scientific and entrepreneurial motivation, relying on funding from venture capitalists to support expensive research and potentially discover marketable applications—and by marketable, the implication is *profitable*. Promotion of gene-editing technologies often emphasizes their ability to eliminate a range of health conditions "lumped together as curable pathologies."[57] The biochemist Jennifer Doudna, who worked on CRISPR, has written about its "potential genetic cures" for things like "achondroplasia (dwarfism), chronic granulomatous disease, Alzheimer's disease, congenital hearing loss, amyotrophic lateral sclerosis (ALS), high cholesterol, diabetes, Tay-Sachs, skin disorders, fragile X syndrome, and even infertility."[58] As Estreich explains, a wide range of conditions are all lumped together as abnormal and framed as forms of "suffering," avoidable or curable through medical interventions. Here's the problem, often overlooked, often silenced: the implied cure entails the elimination of categories of people who dispute the medicalized assumption that their lives are not worth living, that their way of being in the world (without hearing, or with short stature, or with neurodiversity) amounts to tragedy.

Technologies such as NIPT, of course, do not directly alter human genetics, but rather allow for gathering of information about potential genetic conditions. Like earlier forms of prenatal testing, NIPT is often marketed as a tool to identify Down syndrome. And as a for-profit product, it is the subject of extensive marketing, often through websites with educational videos and media coverage that report on people's experiences with NIPT. One test, the MaterniT21 PLUS, references trisomy 21 in its name, and is promoted as an "early risk assessment of Down syndrome and other conditions."[59] It is pushed directly to individual consumers and sold through a rhetoric of personal choice.[60] In general, NIPT is presented to prospective mothers through neutral-sounding language and images, emphasizing risk assessment and the quest for a "healthy" baby. But Down syndrome is often conflated with more severe or health-compromising conditions. Increasingly, in addition to trisomy 21, companies promote NIPT for identifying extremely rare conditions, for which they drastically oversell the accuracy of their tests.[61] The promotional imagery that accompanies NIPT typically includes stereotyped versions of normality: middle-class heterosexual couples, handsome husband and attractive wife, nuclear families set in clean, orderly suburban homes, and babies with no visible disabilities. The marketing sells choice, control, and versions of happiness "equated with certain kinds of bodies and not others."[62] The American Dream.

NIPT doesn't really sell normality; rather, it taps into people's anxiety around health, around the unacknowledged desire to achieve "ideal" families. The power of NIPT both exploits and shapes the desires of consumers.[63] NIPT peddles the promise of control and perfection in an unpredictable world. I never realized how invested I was in the narrow expectations and versions of normality so heavily prized in our society until the days after Michaela was diagnosed with Down syndrome. I was overtaken by a deeply confusing sense of loss, what I now view as a type of misdirected grief. As Tiffani and I left the doctor's office the morning we received the news, we just drove away, initially with no destination in mind. We were adrift. Like the Erikson family when they left Neil behind in California, trying to separate themselves from the anguish of an experience they didn't know how to cope with, we sought some sort of geographic separation from our lives in Menomonie, from the seismic news that had fundamentally rattled our lives. As we drove, we talked. We processed. We cried. We wondered what Michaela's life would be like, and we struggled to imagine an ordinary future.

Will she ever learn to ride a bike? Will she ever drive a car? Will she get married one day? Will she live on her own?

I recognize now that abilities such as riding a bike and driving a car—by no means universal or inherent—are widely celebrated as key milestones in the United States, a culture where personal desires and people's sense of self-identity are thoroughly infused with the values and market logics of consumer capitalism. These milestones tend to represent levels of personal autonomy and independence, particularly in the type of suburban setting where I grew up. Likewise, going to college, getting a job, marriage, owning real estate—these have become benchmarks of middle-class success, empty boxes to check off in the pursuit of happiness narrowly defined as becoming wealthy and shoring up class status. This is the American Dream, as sold to us in advertising, a myth of self-reliance and pull-yourself-up-by-your-bootstraps meritocracy. This is not a recipe for wellbeing, but rather an ideology of material achievement dictated by our economic system and our cultural emphasis on individualism. My loss was not that of a child, but an idea, an unconscious expectation about what it means to be human and what constitutes a supposedly good life.

After having brunch in Eau Claire, after a day of talking and sharing, we drove home, and we began the process of accepting our new world, and, eventually, cultivating a new one.[64]

·   ·   ·   ·   ·

I am not opposed in principle to things like NIPT, to the ability to learn about genetic conditions prenatally, and like Rayna Rapp, I fully support abortion rights. But it simply can't be ignored that NIPT exists in a society where many people, including at one time myself, are heavily invested in cultural values that normalize some types of families and bodies and minds while excluding others. As Estreich writes, "cultural values influence individual decisions, which are, in turn, multiplied by technologies in population effects."[65] Lurking within the sterile language of risk assessment that accompanies prenatal screening technologies is the assumption that Down syndrome represents a deficient existence, an illness to be cured, a misfortune to be avoided.

This assumption results in a population effect: high termination rates of fetuses prenatally diagnosed with trisomy 21, which studies suggest range from 60 to 90 percent in the United States, with significant variation geographically across urban and rural communities, and from 89 to 95 percent in the United Kingdom.[66] In countries with national health care systems such as Denmark, prenatal screening for conditions like Down syndrome occurs in nearly all pregnancies. Most who receive results suggesting that a fetus has Down syndrome pursue abortion. As Sarah Zhang reports for *The Atlantic,* in Denmark "the number of children born with Down syndrome has fallen sharply. In 2019, only 18 were born in the entire country."[67] Prenatal testing, Zhang states bluntly, is changing who does and doesn't get born.

The very desire to screen prenatally for trisomy 21 and these resulting termination rates occur in a cultural context where certain forms of human diversity are stigmatized as undesirable or perceived as burdensome.[68] Routine screening on an individual basis adds up, a collective, societal delineating of normalcy though the systematic "disposal and exclusion of some forms of life," namely, life with Down syndrome.[69] As Rapp observed in the context of amniocentesis in the 1980s and 1990s, the routine use of NIPT to hunt specifically for Down syndrome reinforces its association with "abnormality" or "disease" and positions individuals as moral pioneers not only exercising personal choice, but also acting as the gatekeepers who allow or deny entry into the human community.

It's easy to see the linkages to earlier historical periods when the eugenics movement called explicitly for controlling or limiting the reproduction of certain groups deemed unfit or undesirable, categories of the "feeblemINded" targeted for institutionalization, sterilization, or worse. But now, as disability studies scholar Rosemarie Garland-Thomson puts it, rather than government policy, we are experiencing a kind of "velvet eugenics" achieved through each individual consumer's use of new biomedical technologies, personal decisions informed by "criteria assumed to be reasonable and incontrovertible."[70]

Prenatal testing and the cultural devaluation of Down syndrome does not mean people like my daughter Michaela will disappear from wealthy nations such as the United States, however. In such societies, more people are delaying pregnancy, increasing the statistical likelihood of Down syndrome occurrences. Access to expansive prenatal healthcare is uneven due to racial and class inequalities, and not all will even seek prenatal testing. Among those who do, not everyone will use that information to terminate a pregnancy. With the Supreme Court decision to overturn *Roe v. Wade* in 2022, abortion rights are politically uncertain in the United States and access varies tremendously across the country. Moreover, after decades of disability rights activism, people with Down syndrome are benefiting from healthcare, school, and other support systems, and as a result they are living not only better but also much longer lives. Down syndrome is clearly part of our collective future. Continuing a pregnancy with Down syndrome, however, and, by extension, Down syndrome itself, may increasingly be understood as a personal choice, one stigmatized and devalued, "rather than a socially supported and valuable way of being."[71]

This is the predicament my family now occupies. In 1984, at the dawn of widespread prenatal testing, in the wake of ending her otherwise desired pregnancy, Rapp asked whether such technologies "conflict with our commitment to build a better world for disabled people?" The simple answer is yes, and the troubling reality is that it's not clear whether this conflict is even reconcilable. George Estreich describes this as living simultaneously in two worlds, moving toward two very different futures at the same time. He uses the analogy of home, a space associated with order, security, and the supportive environment of family—but his family's house exists in a liminal, uncertain space, the unknown swirling outside its walls. "It is as if my house were bisected by a border," writes Estreich.

"The front door opens on one country, the back door on another," he says. "In one country [my daughter] is valued and seen, and her difficulties are neither stigmatized, nor held against her, nor used to argue that others like her should not exist; they are accommodated, and she receives what she needs without grudge or pity. In the other country, she is an emblem of the failed pregnancy, a synonym for tragedy, a target of ridicule, an expense to the nation, and the opposite of progress."[72]

This is a paradox of belonging. There is no better time in history than the present moment in which to raise a disabled child, a child such as Michaela who today benefits from decades of struggle for access and accommodation, who is included in school, who finds support and resources in the community, who enjoys access to rights denied to a previous generation. But it is also a moment when others who share her unique chromosomal arrangement are quietly screened for before birth, tested one by one, eliminated through the velvet touch of consumer choice.

The problem, in my view, is not the existence of abortion or prenatal testing, but the cultural values that give meaning to our lives, that inform our expectations and attitudes, that fuel our desire to control reproductive outcomes and seek perfection, however imaginary. These are cultural values that shape our dreams about having certain kinds of children, certain kinds of families, certain kinds of imagined futures. We all indulge in fantasies about what makes life worthwhile, yet most of us rarely pause to stop and question why we are obsessed with achievement, why we define success according to our ability to compete economically, to produce, and to earn money, why we have such a shallow understanding of what makes life meaningful.[73]

Margaret Mead commented on this indirectly in 1969 in a lecture about social change and the generation gap, observing how Americans were projecting expectations, imposing cultural meanings about future success and achievement, onto "the unborn child, already conceived but still in the womb," now a "symbol for what life will be like."

"About the unborn child little can be known with certainty," continued Mead. "No one can know in advance what the child will become—how swift his limbs will be, what will delight his eye, whether his tempo will be fast or slow . . . . No one can know how his mind will work—whether he will learn best from sight or sound or touch or movement. But knowing what we do not know and cannot predict, we can construct an environment in which a child, still unknown, can be safe and can grow and discover himself and the world."[74]

Every Tuesday during the winter, for more than a decade, I've played indoor soccer on the same team in Eau Claire. I love playing soccer, the physical contest, the fast, flowing movement, getting lost in a game and thinking of nothing else. Winning is not the point. I'd rather lose by one goal than win by ten. When the game is close, you are purely and utterly swept up in the moment. Soccer also cultivates a unique camaraderie, bringing together people from all walks of life, longtime residents and recent immigrants, people with wildly differing political beliefs and class backgrounds. None of that matters. I've known guys through soccer for over ten years, and we rarely talk about our lives outside of sport. We have a basic sense of how things are going, but the boundaries are clear. We come together for one type of connection, one shared experience, and that is enough.

I returned home after one relatively late game and Tiffani was already in bed. I made my way upstairs and checked on Aidric and Michaela, both also fast asleep. Then I went into the bathroom for a shower, still high from the euphoria of athletic competition. Reality burst my bubble, or, I should say, the pregnancy test did, a small white dart sitting on the edge of the bathroom sink. Tiffani had left it for me to see.

Michaela was already two and a half years old, and by this point we had settled into our lives. The strangeness of her diagnosis had long faded. She was walking, eating independently, learning to talk through a combination of sign language and vocal utterances, and attending daycare. We recognized a third child would increase the labor of parenting, but it was something we accepted immediately. We were already in parenting mode, had stable, decent-paying jobs, and knew we could welcome a third child into our lives and family. The only question we faced was whether to seek out prenatal screening, such as NIPT.

Increased risk of Down syndrome.

We talked about it, but with no sense of urgency. I even accompanied Tiffani to an appointment with an obstetrician, who explained that NIPT would yield little information about the general health of the fetus that couldn't be gleaned through ultrasounds and other routine prenatal care. It would do nothing to inform any necessary care after its birth. It would do nothing to change the pregnancy. So, we declined, and Tiffani went back to the family physician who had delivered Michaela. Tiffani had one or two ultrasounds during the pregnancy, and as with Aidric and Michaela, we also asked not to be told the gender. Biology means little outside the cultural meanings we assign it.

Months later, Zora arrived on a warm, summer morning, and, sitting alongside her mom and brother, Michaela held her sister for the first time.

6 Vulnerability

As it did for other children across the world, the COVID-19 pandemic transformed Michaela's first two years of elementary school. We were excited for her to go to school, to make friends, to be a part of the community—to make good on the years of struggle by others before her that ensure children with Down syndrome are included. She began kindergarten in the fall of 2020 wearing a face mask and remaining six feet from others, learning new rituals of hand washing and adding "Covid test" to her vocabulary—a reference to the unpleasant nasal swab.

Prior to that, in the spring of 2020, when she was in preschool, schools in Wisconsin sent kids home during the global wave of abrupt shutdowns. I vividly recall the feelings of dread that accompanied the first weeks of the COVID-19 pandemic, the life-altering change introduced by unprecedented lockdowns and the potential economic doom that followed as "nonessential" businesses and other institutions closed their doors. It felt like society was unraveling. People stockpiled toilet paper and watched the cruel spectacle of the president of the United States downplaying COVID-19 through racist references to the "kung flu," spreading misinformation that undermined his administration's own health experts. As the bodies piled up, first in Wuhan, then Italy, and eventually New York

City and elsewhere, people hurriedly stocked their shelves with canned goods and disinfectants and withdrew cash from banks. As a parent, I felt scared in ways I likely would not have if I were younger and on my own. When children depend on you for their safety, your risk calculus changes. But as the parent of a child with Down syndrome, I also found myself pondering the significance of vulnerability. Some people run the risk of becoming more disposable than others.

The UW-Stout campus closed as well. Suddenly, we were all home, an obliteration of normal, Tiffani and I trying to work while supervising three young children. It was a drastic and hellish change. Aidric was in first grade at the time, and his teacher sent home some class materials and tried to host sessions over videoconference. We did our best to maintain some semblance of continuity with his education, to work on reading and math and whatever else, but it was difficult. With his younger sisters home too, there was little in the way of quiet study time. I was suddenly teaching my own courses from our makeshift bedroom office, using videoconference platforms while trying to keep my students engaged amid the upheaval to everyone's lives. My students rarely turned on their cameras and I often found myself lecturing to an essentially blank computer monitor, tiny boxes listing the names of students presumably on the other side. Zora despised being locked out of the room when Tiffani or I needed to work, and she would lay outside the door and relentlessly bang on it with her feet.

The first summer following the initial 2020 pandemic lockdowns, we largely kept to ourselves, diligently social distancing, postponing visits with extended family, avoiding events and gatherings. I took to bike riding with the kids. At first, we even avoided playgrounds, unsure as to whether the virus could spread through interaction with contaminated playground equipment or a chance encounter with another kid. We spent time at soccer fields and rode to lakes and rivers where we could fish or hike. Over time we developed a better understanding of the transmission risks. It became clear that the virus did not readily spread through touching surfaces, and that being outside greatly reduced one's risk of exposure. When the police killed George Floyd in nearby Minneapolis, triggering a new wave of Black Lives Matter protests, we attended a demonstration in town. We started visiting playgrounds again, much to my children's delight, and eventually visited every playground in Menomonie. We loved riding to Wakanda Park with its giant slides and playground equipment among towering trees, the mysterious indigenous burial mound at the edge of a bluff overlooking Lake Menomin.

As the fall 2020 school year approached following six months of lockdowns, I was filled with anxiety and uncertainty. The virus had not waned as many initially expected, and a vaccine still seemed a distant dream. Many large urban school districts around the country were organizing for remote learning or developing hybrid models to greatly reduce the density of kids in classrooms. My own university pursued a hybrid return to campus with a blend of in-person and online courses. Everyone was required to wear masks, tried to maintain six feet from others, sanitized desks, and hoped for the best. The school district adopted a similar plan, requiring everyone, both students and staff, to wear masks. At that time, rural communities had been spared the worst of the initial COVID-19 surges, and in rural Wisconsin there was little political appetite for keeping schools closed or operating remotely. Many families still opted to homeschool or enrolled their kids in an option for virtual schooling from home, which greatly reduced the numbers planning to attend in person. After our experiences in the spring, these options did not seem viable for us. Both Aidric and Michaela would need constant supervision of their learning, requiring one of us to quit our jobs, and we felt Michaela needed the structure and stimulation of interacting with her teachers and peers. It seemed like an awful gamble, but we sent the kids back to school that fall, and Michaela started kindergarten donning a face mask.

I didn't think it would last, fearing that bringing kids together in school and having college students back on campus would seed community-wide outbreaks. But it seemed to work, at least in schools. Community transmission did increase, with a significant fall and winter surge. To the relief of many parents, however, the initial COVID-19 variants were less transmissible among children and the layered mitigation strategies used at schools were surprisingly effective. No outbreaks occurred at Michaela and Aidric's elementary school, nor at Zora's daycare on campus. Only a few cases appeared in the younger elementary school grades the entire year. Michaela's class had one positive case and the entire class had to quarantine for several days. But that was it, a minor disruption in the big scheme of things. At the start of 2021, highly effective vaccines were being rolled out at record pace among adults and things seemed hopeful. By summer of 2021, the virus was in retreat and a post-pandemic world appeared on the horizon.

Hope can be ephemeral, though. In the pandemic's second year, I began to grasp how social conditions contribute to individual vulnerability. Any early sense of a collective, solidarity-based, "we're all in this together" response had faded. Just as children like Michaela benefit from social supports and programs that foster inclusion, systems that bring them into the whole, as Margaret Mead put it, society still has a way of exposing certain groups to avoidable hardships, deeming them expendable in the face of a collective threat.

. . . . .

Although the worldwide spread of a dangerous virus appears universal, certain people face much higher risk of severe illness and death. Age was an early risk factor, especially in the initial dark months of the pandemic, with the elderly and medically frail much more likely to succumb to the disease. During the first waves, children rarely became infected, and even with the Delta variant in 2021, death seemed a rare outcome for kids. But as COVID-19 ravaged nursing homes and hospitalized scores of people over sixty years old, it also worked its way through the foundations of inequality in American society, subjecting marginalized groups to a new form of collective violence.

When societal inequality damages a person's health, medical anthropologists such as Paul Farmer call this "structural violence," a term that offers one way "of describing social arrangements that put individuals and populations in harm's way." These arrangements "are structural because they are embedded in the political and economic organization of our social world; they are violent because they cause injury to people."[1]

The pandemic immediately exposed the fault lines of vulnerability in the structures of U.S. society. In the first several weeks of the pandemic, for example, significant outbreaks occurred at food processing plants, such as the huge Smithfield pork factory in Sioux Falls, South Dakota, which became an early epicenter, with over a thousand cases by April

2020. The plant's workforce embodies recent immigration and refugee history, with workers speaking more than eighty languages and originating from countries throughout Africa, East Asia, and Latin America.[2] At such plants, workers labor for long hours slicing, deboning, and packing the cuts of meat that wealthier, more privileged Americans crave. As some industries went into lockdown to stem infection, food plant workers were deemed essential, and many lacked the means to stay home anyway. Workers of color risked their lives so that other people, safely isolating, likely White and much wealthier, could have meals safely delivered to their homes or enjoy the convenience of curbside pickup.[3]

Similar scenarios played out in cities across the United States: certain groups disproportionately occupied "front line" jobs that could not be conducted remotely. During the first year of the pandemic, densely populated cities were hit hardest, especially neighborhoods where people resided in multigenerational, working-class households, or lived far away from testing sites and healthcare providers. Clear patterns were taking shape. If you were Black, Hispanic, or Native American, you were at much higher risk for infection and death from COVID-19. As of late September 2020, people identifying as White constituted roughly 61 percent of the U.S. population, but only 51 percent of COVID-19 deaths and 44.5 percent of reported infections. Black Americans, by contrast, constituted 12.3 percent of the population but 21.1 percent of deaths and 18.7 percent of infections.[4] People of color carried the heaviest burden of exposure risk, severity of illness, and likelihood of death.[5]

As the pandemic stretched into its second year, the contours of vulnerability continued to shift and evolve, structural violence manifesting across other geographies of inequality. Many big cities, with their large public sector workforces and centralized policymaking authority, often governed by Democratic mayors, maintained strict COVID-19 mitigation practices, requiring use of face coverings indoors and incentivizing or even mandating vaccination of public employees. In my community, by contrast, the only institutions with a consistent mask requirement were the local hospital and the university. Otherwise, mask use indoors was sparse. Vaccination rates lagged, and like masks, vaccination became a contentious, politically partisan issue. In the fall of 2021, the more contagious Delta variant churned through less densely populated areas, which tended to have fewer safety measures in place. Rural counties in Wisconsin have populations that trend older, less healthy, and more economically insecure. This translates into higher rates of death and suffering from COVID-19. By November 2021, the rate of death in rural areas of the United States was double that of urban areas.[6]

Beyond the crossroads of race, class, and place, vulnerability is also structured by gender and disability. During the first several months of the COVID-19 pandemic, for example, the disease swept through many nursing homes in the United States, which were described by some observers as "death pits," language that echoes the critiques of institutionalization in the 1960s and 1970s.[7] Group homes and facilities that provide care for adults with intellectual disabilities were similarly devastated by the virus, with residents becoming infected and dying at far higher rates than the general population.[8] In addition to residents, workers at such facilities, and those who provide home health and personal care services, also faced heightened risk. Most workers in the care work economy that allows people with disabilities to live independently or pursue a dignified life in group home settings are women, and commonly women of color.[9]

.   .   .   .   .

As we approached the fall of 2021 and the second full school year of the COVID-19 pandemic, the community we live in longed for normality. "Birthday treats are back!" announced an email to parents, the quintessential childhood ritual. School officials informed parents their kids could bring treats to share on their birthday. But with one stipulation—only if they were nut-free. "A student has a life-threatening reaction to air-borne peanut products," school officials explained.

As I read, I recalled an ethnographic account of the Dobe Ju/'hoansi of southern Africa, traditionally a foraging society in which the sharing of resources and cooperation are the bedrock for collective success, life organized around kinship-based exchange networks, people working together to subsist in the Kalahari Desert. The Ju/'hoansi do not pay attention to birthdays, do not define personhood in terms of individual uniqueness.[10] The individual is downplayed in favor of the group. In the United States, by contrast, birthday rituals teach children that individualism reigns supreme. *You are part of a community, but you are unique, you are special, you are set apart from the rest.*

Despite the hope that the summer of 2021 would mark the end of the pandemic and restoration of normalcy, warning signs loomed. During the spring, as COVID-19 vaccines became more widely available in the United States, the Delta variant ravaged India and then spread around the world. It appeared to be significantly more transmissible, including among children and the fully vaccinated. Tiffani and I had gotten vaccinated as soon as we were eligible and waited eagerly for the vaccine to be approved for younger children, which would not come for several more months. In the meantime, over the summer the school district had lifted their mask requirement and ended other mitigation protocols. As August approached, though, COVID-19 rates began to rebound, triggering a surge destined to collide with the start of the 2021 school year. We nervously watched these developments, knowing that vaccination rates in our largely rural county were below the national average, and far below recommended thresholds for blunting a return of new COVID-19 variants. But while the school was sending out announcements about the return of birthday treats, we heard nothing about COVID-19 mitigation, such as masks.

Political circumstances in Wisconsin had changed during the second year of the pandemic. In contrast to the previous year, the state government had shifted the responsibility of making public health decisions to local school boards. In the spring of 2021, the conservative-leaning state supreme court had stripped the governor of the authority to mandate masking and other public health safety measures.[11] Further restricting state efforts, the Republican-dominated legislature generally followed the lead of President Trump in its response to the pandemic. During 2020, Trump notoriously downplayed COVID-19 mitigation measures. After being treated for the disease in late 2020, he emerged from his hospitalization in a dramatic appearance on a White House balcony and then defiantly removed his mask, despite still being infectious, solidifying unmasking as a political symbol for his supporters. Following the lead of Trump during his embattled final year in the presidency, Wisconsin legislators from the Republican party similarly opposed masks and other mitigation strategies. By the summer of 2021, the state government was limited in its authority to do much of anything, other than issue recommendations.

Local municipalities and school districts were left to set their own policies.

In the absence of state public health rules, the county health department provided its recommendations to the school board. The county we live in is politically divided and leans conservative, and beyond Menomonie, a small city of roughly sixteen thousand people, it is largely rural. The county government and public health department lacked the political will and capacity to issue or enforce mandates. In line with federal and state recommendations, they merely advised the school district to require universal masking of students and staff, regardless of vaccination status, given the contagious Delta variant.[12] This was also recommended by the school district's own medical advisor. Even the district superintendent supported a mask requirement, emphasizing that it would keep kids in school and reduce the likelihood that they would face quarantines or other disruptions to their education.

The school board, however, appeared set to ignore these recommendations, and moved to start the school year without masks, the linchpin of a layered mitigation strategy. As we prepared for Michaela to start first grade, we faced a dilemma. Our children were still too young to be vaccinated, unable to access the most effective mitigation strategy available. Plus, over the first eighteen months of the COVID-19 pandemic, more was being learned about the increased vulnerability of people with Down syndrome, which by then had been listed by the Centers for Disease Control and Prevention as a risk category for severe illness. Children with Down syndrome tend to do better than adults, but researchers were looking at how the genetic implications of that extra chromosome contributed to the increased risk.[13] Down syndrome is often associated with a higher rate of preexisting health conditions, such as heart issues. Even when these don't exist, respiratory problems and immune system issues are more common among people with Down syndrome. A study in late 2020 found that people with Down syndrome who got COVID-19 were four times more likely to be hospitalized, and ten times more likely to die, than the general population.[14]

In some ways, fate was on Michaela's side in her early years, sparing her any health complications related to her extra chromosome. She also benefited from all the privileges of a White middle-class family and the support systems available in our community. But at the interface of biology and society, vulnerability changes and contorts as life unfolds, shaped by conditions far beyond our control. Tiffani and I pondered everything we had learned about COVID-19 and the unique risk factors facing children with Down syndrome and agonized over whether school would be safe for her. We also expected that approval of the vaccine for her age group was just around the corner. If we could just hold out a little longer, she would have access to a powerful vaccine and the protection it offers.

August brought a flurry of school board meetings focused on possibly restoring mitigation measures. Hundreds of parents attended, with many opposing mask requirements. I knew masks were unpopular in rural Wisconsin, but I hadn't anticipated the passionate expressions of deep, bitter resentment. A large antimask contingent cheered on fellow critics and loudly jeered at anyone who spoke in support of mitigation measures, angrily mocking the school district medical advisor and threatening the county public health director. It wasn't just masks—they opposed any sort of COVID-19 mitigation measures at school. One person compared public health officials to Nazis.

An argument certainly existed for not mandating masks in schools.[15] Only rarely, however, did the speakers who attended the embattled school board meetings attempt to address the efficacy of masks, and they typically did so by denying the validity of medical science, not debating the issues based on competing forms of evidence. It was a typical "denialist playbook" used to advance purely rhetorical arguments.[16] A dentist, for example, introduced himself as a doctor to exaggerate his own claim to expertise, and then argued that masks are only effective in clinical settings. This was joined by comments from other people who raised doubts about the severity of the COVID-19 pandemic or downplayed the risk among children, selectively citing all manner of superficial data. Several people described the evolving scientific understanding of COVID-19 to assert that concern about the pandemic was overblown, magnifying expected disagreements among scientists trying to understand a new disease. A few denied the pandemic's existence outright. Several people raised the specter of vaccine mandates, suggesting that mitigation measures such as mask requirements were just a step closer to government biopolitical control. Many others emphasized parent choice, asserting that they alone should have a say about the healthcare decisions of their children. Some warned against government decrees and cast public health officials as part of a scheme to take away people's freedoms. One person screamed that their child had an "immune system, and it [was] strong, and natural immunity" would keep her safe.

Amid the strife of public commentary for or against masks, I spoke at three different board meetings, and offered a unique perspective. I explained that Michaela can attend public school only because of decades of civil rights struggles. Barely fifty years ago, children like her were just as likely to end up segregated in special institutions, subject to potential abuse and neglect, as to attend neighborhood schools. Their parents fought to gain access to schools, community-based services, and other opportunities. Federal law protects her right to a free appropriate public education in the least restrictive environment, setting into motion structures and supports, enabling the hiring of teachers, therapists, and aides, a system that ensures a place for Michaela alongside her peers.[17] Because of these laws, children with Down syndrome are now included in their communities in ways once unimaginable.

With the Delta variant ripping through western Wisconsin and given the clear public health consensus about how to keep kids safe, it was difficult to see how universal masking in schools, at least temporarily, could be interpreted as anything but reasonable. Just like any other student, Michaela has a right to access a safe learning environment along with her peers. The school board, I argued, by declining to follow the guidance of their own medical advisors and district leadership, would be violating my daughter's right to safely go to school.[18] In fact, the U.S. Department of Education had recently announced civil rights investigations in five states that prohibited indoor masking in schools because such policies appeared to discriminate against students with disabilities.[19]

My argument, however, went nowhere. Two days before the start of school, the school board opted once again to oppose COVID-19 mitigation, voting 5–4 in favor of "optional" masking—*optional* being the equivalent of nothing. The board voted to ignore the recommendations of federal and state public health agencies, of county health officials, of district leadership, and of its own medical advisor. Children at increased risk, such as Michaela, could choose to wear a mask, or they could choose to stay home.

I found it disturbing that a group of people with no medical expertise had the authority to disregard health officials and create policy that undermines student safety, a situation that played out in rural communities across Wisconsin and the United States. For many community members who spoke at the board meetings and had the ear of the school board, pseudo-expertise and defense of individual liberties mixed with a distrust of government institutions and outright conspiracy theory. The ensuing fog of selective vision and self-deception made reasoned, evidence-based debate impossible. In place of debate, a spectacle had unfolded in which people articulated starkly different worldviews. In one of those worldviews, COVID-19 mitigation signaled a threat to individual liberty. Personal choice had become survival of the fittest.

What is also striking is how easily disability rights were ignored or dismissed. In that peculiar historical moment, a uniquely American carnage, our society grew callous to several hundred thousand deaths nationwide (over 1 million deaths by May 2022, a far higher death rate than any other wealthy country), along with the suffering of countless others. In the email about the return of birthday treats, food allergies had elicited appeals for collective action, yet children with disabilities or other medical vulnerabilities remained expendable. Food allergies are certainly serious, something a child has no control over. It makes sense to ask others to endure small sacrifices so that everyone has access to a safe learning environment at school, allowing all children the opportunity to develop and flourish, without risking their lives. At the end of the day, we are all responsible to each other. But while birthday treats were back, the classic expression of American individualism, COVID-19 mitigation was not. The indifference sanctioned by the school board was bolstered by the outright hostility of many parents. The same parents who would otherwise comply with requests to protect the anonymous kid with nut allergies passionately refused to send their child to school with a mask.

The day before school started, we made the agonizing decision to keep Michaela out of school, Tiffani taking an unpaid leave of absence to stay home with her. Aidric, though, expressed a strong desire to attend in person, so we sent him and implored him to wear his mask. Zora, too, went to her 4K program at the campus daycare, which had a mask requirement and strictly enforced other safety measures. Weeks later, COVID-19 cases predicably increased in the community and in the schools, leading to a skyrocketing number of students being excluded due to quarantine requirements. Given the opportunity to revisit their decision, the school board doubled down, once again disregarding expert advice from public health officials and medical doctors, deciding instead to make quarantine optional too.

Several weeks later, as the situation with COVID-19 deteriorated in the schools and community, we found ourselves at the center of a larger conflict over public health and disability rights, initiating legal action against a school board for their failure to follow basic recommendations to keep children safe at school.

.   .   .   .   .

That, during a global health emergency, others in my community view masks as unnecessary or vaccines as potentially dangerous is not a question of political difference or even professional training, but one of belief. At its extreme, it reflects a rejection of science, and at best a dangerous loss of trust in public health experts. The school board members who voted against requiring masks had only laypeople's understanding of the issues. Their rationales for ignoring public health recommendations were typically based on the symbolic meaning of masks in a divisive political climate, not on the efficacy of specific mitigation strategies. They were emboldened by beliefs gaining traction within a significant cross-section of the community, beliefs that enabled them to rationalize ignoring the advice of the school district's own expert medical advisors, with potentially grave consequences.

Some scholars trace the beliefs that coalesced around the issue of masking to a longstanding "health freedom movement" with deep historical roots in the United States. During the nineteenth century, efforts to create licensing statutes in the medical field provoked opposition from "drugless practitioners" including "mind-curers, Christian Scientists, and osteopaths," as well as other allies of alternative medicines.[20] The first antivaccine leagues were created in the nineteenth century, and protest of smallpox inoculations can be traced back even further. In the early twentieth century, popular movements for "freedom of therapeutic choice" continued to challenge state laws that sought to create standards for the medical establishment, maintaining a space for alternative healers and challenging public health initiatives such as vaccination laws.[21]

As the boundaries and standards of medical expertise formalized over the twentieth century, and with increased public trust in science and medicine following World War II, alternative medicine movements were pushed to the fringes of society.[22] After the polio pandemic of 1949–52, which left some infected children with paralyzed muscles and disfigured limbs, the advent of a polio vaccine in 1954 found widespread support among parents. As medical doctor and vaccine specialist Peter Hotez explains, this was followed by "a string of successes in the development of new vaccines against measles, mumps, rubella, *Haemophilus influenzae* type B, and rotavirus, among others."[23] Childhood vaccination mandates triggered some backlash, but by 1980 all fifty states required vaccination among schoolchildren.[24]

According to Hotez, an interlinking of interest in sensationalized cures, the growth of supplement and natural foods industries, and skepticism of government helped revitalize health freedom politics in the early twenty-first century, eventually colliding with the COVID-19 pandemic. "Its two major tenets included access to nontraditional medications or supplements, and opposition to traditional health practices."[25] Around the 1970s, ideas associated with health freedom found expression in a range of sometimes disparate causes that unfolded into the early 2000s: New Age philosophies and spiritual movements; critique of multinational pharmaceutical companies and corporate control of food systems; suspicion of genetically modified foods; political opposition to regulation of supplements, vitamins, and natural products; legalization of medical marijuana; access to experimental treatments for AIDS in the 1980s; access to abortion; legalization of physician-assisted suicide; and expansion of alternative treatments within orthodox medicine, among others.[26]

Vaccines would come to embody the intersection of claims about freedom from government regulation with access to alternative and so-called "natural" health treatments, boosted by a late 1990s controversy. In 1998,

The Lancet published a paper by British medical doctor Andrew Wakefield and several colleagues that asserted a relationship between the measles-mumps-rubella vaccine and diagnosis of autism in children, which exploited a widespread fear of cognitive disability and "ushered in a new era of distrust for vaccine."[27] Autism, or autism spectrum disorder, describes a complex condition or form of neurodiversity that can manifest behaviorally in many ways. Increasing rates of diagnosis in the 1990s fueled unfounded worries of an "autism epidemic," even though the supposed increase reflected evolving diagnostic definitions and the growth of efforts to identify and provide services to people with developmental disabilities. As anthropologist Roy Grinker argues, there was never an autism epidemic, only an increase in diagnosis and an intensifying cultural impulse to medically categorize forms of behavior that seemed to fall outside conceptions of normality.[28] Wakefield's paper, however, despite eventually being exposed as fraudulent and withdrawn from *The Lancet,* tapped into deeper anxieties about the specter of disability and impairment.

Wakefield himself was discredited and banished from Britain's medical profession, but the damage was done. He moved to the United States and continued to insist on the linkage and advocate against vaccines. Vaccine hesitancy among parents grew through online publications and fringe forums, with some parents adopting health freedom rhetoric and invoking religious or personal exemptions to avoid vaccinating their school-aged children. Such actions found support among alternative medicine practitioners, including some who have a veneer of legitimacy, such as chiropractors. Isolated measles outbreaks, including the 2014–15 outbreak in Orange County, California, prompted efforts in some states to remove such exemptions, which in turn invigorated grassroots opposition and invited allegations of a government-medical-corporate ploy to push vaccines. Once considered eliminated in the United States, measles surged; cases exceeded a thousand in 2019 as conservative states maintained or created parent exemptions to school vaccination requirements.[29] As Hotez describes, opponents "implemented a system of pseudoscience claiming that vaccines were toxic, or that natural immunity acquired from the illness was superior and more durable than vaccine-induced immunity," and antivaccine organizations and political action committees formed in many states to bolster such assertions.[30]

Antivaccine groups were already organized and primed to react when the COVID-19 pandemic hit, their rhetoric churning amid the fraught context of the final year of the Trump administration, which nurtured white nationalist views, cast doubt on scientific expertise, elevated conspiracy theories, and cultivated distrust of government institutions. The cringe-worthy ruminations of President Trump about COVID-19 miracle cures, even ingesting bleach, gave expression to and amplified beliefs circulating as part of a once-scattered health freedom movement.[31]

As summer 2021 approached, COVID-19 appeared to be in retreat, and the newly elected administration of President Joe Biden planned to celebrate a symbolic reopening of society. The Delta variant, however, ushered in a new phase of sickness and death. The Biden administration responded by encouraging corporations to mandate vaccines among their workers and by announcing new vaccine requirements for federal employees and contractors. The possibility of vaccine mandates invigorated antivaccine activism, which continued to mutate with the evolving pandemic. Longstanding strands of health freedom activism became a dangerous source of antiscience misinformation, fueling local, grassroots activism that emphasized personal choice and so-called natural immunity as the only acceptable responses to a global pandemic, viewing public health policy as a form of tyrannical government overreach.[32]

Claims about building natural immunity, articulated at our school board meetings in Menomonie, invoke the modern image of the pliable "immune system," binding it to deeply held cultural beliefs. As anthropologist Emily Martin analyzed in her 1994 book *Flexible Bodies*, the then-new discourse of immunity adheres closely to cultural values of personal responsibility and individual choice, finding expression through narratives of building health through diet, exercise, and spiritual growth. This image of the immune system is curiously consistent with the dominant values of a capitalist society: individual self-empowerment and cutthroat competition in the pursuit of personal gain and profit.

In the context of the COVID-19 pandemic, such immune system discourse was mobilized to oppose masks and vaccines, to undermine collective, solidarity-based responses to a societal crisis. Public health policy was perceived as an attack on individual "corporeal freedom."[33] As Martin warned decades ago, this all has the contours of a new social Darwinism, a survival-of-the-fittest mentality echoing the eugenics movement of the early twentieth century.[34]

.   .   .   .   .

After the COVID-19 vaccine was approved and as the hopefulness of summer 2021 deteriorated into a new wave of illness, Wisconsin's budding health freedom movement found institutional support among chiropractors. The chiropractic profession has a peculiar history, with nineteenth-century roots in alternative medicine and beliefs in almost supernatural innate life forces. Over the course of the twentieth century, it has often been criticized as a medical quackery.[35] During the COVID-19 pandemic, a split in the profession saw some chiropractors emerge as a source of vocal and energetic vaccine skepticism. With degrees from chiropractic schools that award the title of doctorate to their graduates, chiropractors lent a gloss of medical credibility to the claims of health freedom activists.

In April 2021, the Chiropractic Society of Wisconsin (CSW) hosted Vax-Con '21 in the Wisconsin Dells, billed as an educational opportunity where practitioners could receive continuing education credits. A relatively new player on the scene, the CSW formed in 2012 to lobby against state licensing standards for chiropractors. It was established as a rival to the longstanding Wisconsin Chiropractic Association (WCA), founded in 1911. Both associations engage in significant political lobbying, but in 2021 the CSW became an organizational force behind antivaccine efforts in the state, promoting misinformation about the COVID-19 vaccines and coordinating with national and international antivaccine groups. Vax-Con '21 was a sold-out event that pushed misinformation, featuring prominent antivaccine activists as keynote speakers, including the star of the 2020 viral conspiracy video "Plandemic: The Hidden Agenda behind COVID-19," which was viewed millions of times on YouTube.[36]

In the summer and fall of 2021, the CSW also hosted a series of Health Freedom Revival events in rural Wisconsin. Speakers included the California-based chiropractor Billy DeMoss, who prior to the pandemic was raising money through an event called Cal Jam for antivaccine groups such as Children's Health Defense. DeMoss advertised his appearance at the Health Freedom Revival in a characteristically flamboyant social media video while wearing a black hat and t-shirt, both emblazoned with the phrase "COVID IS A SCAM."[37] Such gestures mark the health freedom movement's cross-fertilization of antiscience misinformation, COVID-19 denialism, and vaccine skepticism.

The Health Freedom Revivals also featured Nebraska-based chiropractor Ben Tapper, listed by the Center for Countering Digital Hate in 2021 as among a "dirty dozen" leading online social media influencers who spread conspiracy theories and vaccine misinformation.[38] In their social media promotion, the CSW described Tapper as a doctor who "serves the community in health, including the vax injured," advocating for "true health and the bodies [sic] innate ability to heal." Mystical ideas of innate healing forces tie together notions of holistic medicine, self-improvement, and vague claims about supernatural regenerative qualities. Speakers such as Tapper are framed as experts through reference to doctorates from chiropractic schools, making them seem like a legitimate source of medical advice. This gesture toward expert status accompanies a conspiracy-laden rejection of mainstream medicine and science, framed as threats to personal health and liberty.[39]

The warped messages churning out of the health freedom movement are clear: denialism of COVID-19, a global pandemic that has spread sickness and death to millions around the world; conspiracy theories about vaccines as part of a medical-government-corporate experiment, rather than an effective tool to tame disease; fear of public health as an oppressive force eroding individual rights, rather than an effort to mobilize a collective response to a societal challenge; criticism of masks and vaccines as threats to bodily integrity and autonomy, with true health only possible through personal empowerment, a strong immune system, and cultivation of inner spiritual forces. As anthropologist Susannah Crockford explains, the health freedom movement ironically "casts vaccination as eugenics," a form of "population control aimed at the most vulnerable for the profit of healthcare and pharmaceutical corporations. Their rhetoric positions them as the underdog fighting for freedom against the oppressor."[40]

Such views are not merely the fodder of remote, revivalist gatherings, but also find expression among state lawmakers, and, of course, local school boards. In the summer of 2021, our local state assemblyman, Clint

Moses, a chiropractor by profession who at the time also served on the school board, was the lead coauthor of proposed Assembly Bill 309, which sought to "prohibit discrimination based on vaccination status." Moses has been supported by the CSW and was featured at the Health Freedom Revivals along with DeMoss, Tapper, and other peddlers of disinformation. With some cities in the United States requiring proof of vaccination for various activities and with numerous companies requiring vaccination among employees, the proposed bill sought to include "vaccination status" as a protected category under state antidiscrimination laws, specifically calling out provisions that require accommodations or protections for people with disabilities to justify the bill. Created to protect one of the most marginalized and stigmatized groups in society, disability rights were instead being invoked as part of a health freedom movement aligned with vaccine skeptics, conspiracy theorists, and opponents of public health. In testimony given before the proposed bill eventually failed, Moses described COVID-19 vaccines as "experimental therapy." He suggested that people were being "shamed" for not wearing a mask or being vaccinated, and that as a "healthcare provider" he wanted to protect them from such prejudice.[41]

.   .   .   .   .

Such rhetoric was echoed by the public comments made at our local school board meetings, some of them equating public health to authoritarianism. Our school board was receptive to these attitudes, ignoring all levels of medical recommendations to keep kids safe, drawing on the same swirl of beliefs and rationales associated with the health freedom movement to justify their decision.

Many other school boards in Wisconsin, especially in rural areas, did the same. Then, barely a month into the school year, the first student death linked to COVID-19 was reported in a Wisconsin school district with no mask requirement. A thirteen-year-old middle school student in Fort Atkinson died unexpectedly after having had a mild cold for two days. He was later found to be positive for COVID-19. The Fort Atkinson school board quickly changed course and voted to require masks, which had been optional.[42] If that wasn't devastating enough, a few days later a seventeen-year-old student at Mondovi High School died from pneumonia-related complications after testing positive for COVID-19. This second death struck close to home for the Menomonie school board, since Mondovi is scarcely a forty-minute drive south, located in a neighboring county. A week later, that board also changed course and began requiring masks in schools.[43]

Amid all of this, Tiffani and I made the difficult decision to retain a lawyer with the intent to file a legal action against the school board on the basis that their decision not to implement public health recommendations effectively denied Michaela equal access to a free and appropriate public education. Retaining a lawyer was a difficult decision because we had no desire to be the parents who "sued" their school district, nor to put ourselves at the center of the controversy surrounding masks. Legal counsel is also extraordinary expensive, so we initially hesitated. But as COVID-19 cases increased and the school board responded by making quarantine optional, further reducing COVID-19 mitigation, we also temporarily pulled Aidric from school and felt we had no choice but to take some sort of legal action.

Coincidentally, the day we decided to retain a lawyer, a proposal for masking was again put on the school board agenda, a response to the two recent student deaths in Wisconsin. I didn't expect it to pass, but the new mask proposal was framed as a compromise. The mask requirement would apply only to students who were not yet eligible to become vaccinated, those in kindergarten through sixth grade. In this framing, these students and their parents were denied a "choice" to become vaccinated. The local media had also learned that a Menomonie family was preparing legal action, though we had not yet gone public, but the news report added to the pressure on the board.[44] In addition, dozens of teachers organized to speak out at the board meeting, requesting a mask requirement. The discourse of parental choice, combined with the recent student deaths, the specter of legal action, and the mobilization of teachers, resonated with one of the five antimask board members, who surprisingly flipped their vote and supported the compromise. The partial student mask requirement passed 5–4.

I was truly relieved. I assumed we would not need to make good on having retained a lawyer, saving us the several thousand-dollar retainer fee that I had put on a credit card only the day before. With the mask requirement in place, Aidric returned to school after nearly two weeks at home. We also decided to send Michaela back, reasoning that if the school was at least adopting recommended mitigation measures, attending school in person justified the risk. Before doing so, however, we initiated communications with her school, seeking a guarantee that the teachers and staff who work closely with her would wear masks, and inquiring about the vaccination status of staff who would interact closely with her. But a few hours after hitting send on that email to the school, we learned that the school board was already backpedaling. Presumably coming under tremendous pressure, the board initiated a special board meeting for the following Sunday afternoon, where they would reconsider the days-old mask requirement. That was the point at which we decided that the school board was not only reckless in its disregard for public health but also unpredictable in its policymaking. We couldn't send Michaela back, even with the mask requirement, without assurance the school board wouldn't rescind its own policies days later.

The next day, our attorney sent the board a letter on our behalf, formally requesting a due process hearing under the Individuals with Disabilities Education Act (IDEA). This law ensures that students like Michaela receive individualized education plans (IEPs) tailored to their unique needs and requires schools to provide reasonable accommodations so that public education is accessible to children with disabilities. The due process hearing is a legal mechanism to resolve disputes within the IEP process. The political circumstances in Wisconsin meant we had few other legal options available. In the absence of state, city, or county mandates, public health guidelines are merely recommendations and school boards have tremendous latitude to set policy. Recent lawsuits in other states had challenged state-level prohibitions on local mask requirements, arguing that such bans violate the rights of students with disabilities by putting them at increased risk. A federal judge ruled, for example, that Texas Governor Greg Abbott's ban on mask mandates in local schools violated the Americans with Disabilities Act.[45] Our situation did not involve a state-level ban on masks, however, but a local school board unwilling to follow the advice of public health officials and its own medical advisors. While the same principle is at stake—*policy creating unsafe conditions that put children with disabilities at risk*—our lawyer opted to take a different legal path. Since we had kept Michaela at home at the last second, the board's failure to adopt appropriate COVID-19 safety policies meant the district was denying her access to a free appropriate education. Our request for a due process hearing specified that to ensure Michaela could exercise her fundamental right to a free appropriate public education, her school must implement a universal mask requirement, ensure staff are vaccinated, enforce the county quarantine policy, and practice social distancing. Basically, we asked that they follow public health recommendations. Moments after sending the letter, our lawyer alerted interested media contacts that the first mask-related legal action had been initiated in Wisconsin.[46] The following day, the special Sunday board meeting was cancelled, without explanation, keeping the mask requirement in place.

This, to me, represented a victory. Without our legal action, the board likely would have rescinded its provisional mask requirement barely a week after it was adopted. Roughly a week later, the school district responded to our request for a due process hearing in a formal letter. They asked us to withdraw our legal action, since a mask mandate was now in place. As I sat pondering whether we could really have faith in the school board sticking to its policy, a few hours later the agenda for the next board meeting was published. Removing the mask requirement was once again on the agenda! The district knew this was coming, even as they pressured us to withdraw our legal action. The agenda item was accompanied by an extraordinary statement: "this proposal [to make masking optional] is not aligned with the recommendations of the Centers for Disease Control, the Wisconsin Department of Health Services, the Dunn County Health Department, the [district] Medical Advisors, the [...] District Administrator, the [district] Administrative Team, the district's liability insurance carrier, and the advice of [district] legal counsel."

If there was any doubt that our legal action was operating to keep the board from removing the mask requirement, it became clear during the actual board meeting, when the board chair cited legal jeopardy as their rationale for voting to keep the requirement in place. This happened again weeks later, after the COVID-19 vaccine was approved for children five to eleven years old in early November 2021. Immediately, the board proposed to remove the mask requirement, even though it would be several weeks before those interested in the vaccine could get the two doses to be considered fully vaccinated. Again, the board chair refused to support lifting the requirement, citing our legal action. Our action was operating as a stopgap mechanism keeping masking in place, at least in the elementary schools. In the meantime, though, with these persistent efforts to eliminate the mask requirement, Michaela remained at home as we waited for the due process hearing. From our perspective, the district's actions were excluding her. Our fight to defend her rights, however, was benefiting others.

Many other parents expressed their appreciation and contributed to a fund to sustain our legal action, a powerful show of solidarity in a context where the health freedom movement was emphasizing survival of the fittest. The legal process unfolded slowly and remained unresolved even as Michaela became fully vaccinated and returned to school. Part of our dispute was resolved through a settlement, the district agreeing to provide afterschool tutoring to make up what Michaela had missed out on when she remained home. Amid the slow-moving legal process, the COVID-19 pandemic then saw yet another turning point, as the Omicron variant quickly supplanted Delta and fueled skyrocketing infections across the United States.

The due process hearing was finally held in early 2022, and centered on whether the school was obligated to follow public health guidelines to ensure accessibility to children like Michaela. But for legal purposes, the judge overseeing the hearing was narrowly focused on Michaela's individual circumstances: a vaccinated, otherwise healthy kid with Down syndrome, who at that point was again attending school in person. The school district brought in an internationally renowned expert witness to argue that it is safe for a vaccinated child with Down syndrome to attend school, even in the absence of recommended mitigation measures, and even though he would recommend that Michaela's school follow public health guidelines around masking. Vaccination reduces a child's risk so much, he testified, that at an individual level, masking and other mitigation measures offer little added protection—statistically speaking, for the individual.

Given the narrow focus of the case at hand, the judge ruled in favor of the district. Since we chose to vaccinate her, it was deemed safe for her to attend school, even in the absence of recommended mitigation measures. The irony, of course, is that the school board deliberately ignored medical expertise in its policymaking when it capitulated to the ideology of the health freedom movement, but then relied on that same medical expertise for its defense at our due process hearing.

We shouldn't equate Down syndrome with vulnerability, and disability should not be reduced to physical or cognitive impairments that may or may not have consequences for a person's life or health.[47] Everyone, regardless of the nature of their body or mind, faces vulnerability as a part of being human. As disability studies scholar Tom Shakespeare reminds us, "to be born is to be vulnerable, to fall prey to disease and pain and suffering, and ultimately to die."[48] A mutual, inevitable dependency on the care of others is a basic prerequisite of human existence.[49]

The COVID-19 pandemic is a stark reminder of this. The question is whether other factors combine with that general human vulnerability to put certain groups into the crosshairs of structural violence. The character of the vulnerability one experiences in life is shaped not only by human biology but also by social conditions, including the interfacing of economics and politics with the belief systems through which people rationalize their behaviors or inactions, or justify their disregard for the wellbeing of others.

Amid the historic moment of the COVID-19 pandemic, I realized that to defend my daughter's right to attend school in person, to defend disability rights, aligns us with a broader effort to push back against a dangerous, antiscience social movement that puts all children at increased risk of harm and undermines public health. Ruth Benedict once said the purpose of anthropology is "to make the world safe for human differences." Parenting a child with Down syndrome, I have learned, enrolls you in an ongoing project to build a world where it is not only safe to be different, but where the most vulnerable are safe from structural violence.

Epilogue

Before the end of her life, Margaret Mead had come to understand disability as part of the richness of human diversity. Disability, however, is not merely a form of diversity, just another identity in a multicultural world. It's a fundamental reality of the human experience shared in some way by all of us, manifesting in diverse and complex forms, and often at various stages of the life cycle. Decades later, disability scholars and activists routinely make this argument. "Our bodies need care, we need assistance to live; we are fragile, limited, and pliable in the face of life itself," writes Rosemarie Garland-Thomson, whose work has been foundational in the creation of disability studies as an interdisciplinary academic field. "Disability is thus inherent in our being: what we call disability is perhaps the essential characteristic of being human."[1]

It is a basic truth of the human condition, one that I had failed to understand when Michaela was first born.[2] Perhaps Mead had also misunderstood this when Erik Erikson called her about Neil, a friend reaching out in a moment of crisis. The feelings of rejection, the temptation to dehumanize, the failure to account for disability as human difference. My experience echoes that of Mead and Erikson.

Parenting a child with Down syndrome has brought me into closer proximity with disability in ways I never imagined possible, pushing me to reconsider assumptions about ideas at the core of my profession, and to confront the histories that still influence anthropology in the present. Disability activism and disability studies have grown in influence in recent years, but disability is far from central to anthropology as it is practiced today.[3] There is still work to be done. Acknowledging disability transforms how we consider basic questions about what it means to be human and how we think about the social forces that shape our perception and experience of difference.

Even though we should acknowledge disability as a form of diversity and as inherent to the human condition, we shouldn't lose sight of its particularity or flatten the nuance of unique disability experiences. Definitions of disability change over time and vary across cultures. There is diversity within disability, and the experiences of disabled people, as well as parents and other caretakers, range widely. My story is by no means universal. In some ways, telling it also indulges in the tendency to examine the nondisabled person's response to disability, a father grappling with his reaction to Down syndrome, as if this were the only thing worthy of anthropological attention when it comes to disability. As such, it is only a starting point.

Beyond my profession and similar academic fields, proximity to disability fosters new and deeper recognition of alternative ways to live and cultivate community.[4] This is a project stretching back to the parent advocacy movement of 1950s and continuing with the disability rights movement of the 1970s to the present. Michaela has enrolled me in this movement, and part of me longs for a world in which my daughter's difference fades into the familiar safety of ordinariness, an unremarkable way of being human.

But this is not the world we currently inhabit, at least not beyond our immediate family. I have also come to appreciate this proximity as a predicament, both something "many people have to face in life," as disability scholar Tom Shakespeare puts it—whether that is my great-grandfather using a wheelchair, my grandmother lost to mental illness and institutionalization, or me and my brother's experiences with debilitating anxiety— and something "everyone should think about."[5] The predicament stems from the social and cultural forces working to exclude Michaela, bearing down on her, the forms of prejudice that lurk amid outward claims of accommodation, the social production of vulnerability and structural violence, the coexisting attitudes of inclusion and elimination that inform contemporary views of Down syndrome.

This predicament is simultaneously a creative force. Something Mead also anticipated, and which is less often recognized, is that disability is not just an inevitability of the human experience, but also generative. Disability is a positive, valuable part of many people's lives, a source of innovation and progressive change, a basis for building new forms of solidarity and community, and an important way of being in, knowing, and experiencing the world.[6]

Michaela teaches me this daily. She enriches my life, and my approach to anthropology.

.   .   .   .   .

In the summer of 2022, Michaela is now seven years old. COVID-19 is no longer avoided but managed. Our bike rides to area playgrounds are less frequent, replaced by visits to museums, zoos, and other destinations we had skipped early in the pandemic. These days, the red trailer gathers dust in the garage. Michaela rides her own bike.

The end of the day comes quickly. After swings and slides and climbing and playing tag and visiting the Wakanda Park burial mound and bathroom breaks and water breaks and snacks and kids whining and kids fighting and kids refusing to leave, we ride home. Aidric and Zora zoom ahead, and I ride alongside Michaela.

"We're home," she eventually announces. "This is my home."

Tiffani is back from work and has started preparing dinner. Michaela begs to watch a movie, *WALL-E* or *Moana* or *Raya and the Last Dragon* or *Turning Red*—she loves movies. The kids argue over what to watch but eventually come to an agreement. Food is served. They are picky eaters but still expect dessert. The evening folds into bedtime. I clean up the table but leave the dishwashing for the next day.

Tiffani usually changes the kids into pajamas and helps brush their teeth, and I assist. Then she says goodnight and goes up to our bedroom. I stay with the kids, reading stories and following a routine of saying goodnight and singing two songs, always the same two songs. At the end of it all, I kiss them each goodnight.

The room is dark. I step toward Michaela's bed. She has a special blanket that she gestures for me to put over her. Then I lean down and put my cheek next to hers as she wraps her arms around me.

"Goodnight, Michaela. I love you."

She replies with her butterfly whisper, and then drifts off to sleep.

Acknowledgments

For more than a few years, the idea for this book nagged at the back of my mind, a project that I would get to eventually, and it was nudged along by circumstance. I finally took some time to write a cathartic essay about my experiences, which appeared in *Sapiens: Anthropology Magazine* back in January 2019, titled "A Daughter's Disability and a Father's Awakening." I appreciated the opportunity to write for *Sapiens* and am grateful that the Wenner-Gren Foundation supports public anthropology. I am thankful for the assistance I received from Chip Colwell, Amanda Mascarelli, Aaron Brooks, and others at *Sapiens*.

After that essay was published, it was featured on the *Sapiens* podcast. I soon received an email from Kate Marshall at University of California Press asking whether I was working on a book project. So, I started working on a book project. Such an endeavor would have typically taken me several years, but then the world seemed to unravel, as it does now and then, and the pandemic lockdowns of 2020 halted my other projects and left me to channel my unease into writing (and bike riding). Kate provided crucial feedback and encouragement at several stages as the book manuscript quickly took shape, for which I am immensely grateful. I am also thankful for the comments I received from anonymous reviewers who looked at a partial manuscript, and for the supportive feedback from Aaron Jackson and Chris Kaposy, who also served as reviewers. My colleagues and friends Lopa Basu, Megan Davidson, and Susan Pietrzyk read the full manuscript as well, for which I am grateful. Daniel Renfrew also read the manuscript and, as usual, provided supportive feedback and helpful suggestions. Caroline Knapp was a remarkably astute copyeditor, both thoughtful and caring. Any errors in the book are of course my responsibility, and I hope they are few.

Even though most didn't have a hand in the manuscript itself, I am thankful for support from my colleagues at University of Wisconsin-Stout. Heather Stecklein, an amazing archivist, supported this book by supporting my courses and my students, as did others in the university library who processed all my unusual book and article requests. My colleagues in the social science department make working at Stout worthwhile. Many of them have been around for this entire journey, among them Tina Lee, Nels Paulson, and Chris Ferguson, and we've been together long enough to share in many of life's joys and challenges.

I am by no means the first parent/scholar to traverse much of the terrain covered in this book, so it's important to acknowledge the collective effort of all who came and wrote before me. Much of their work is cited in or found its way into my book. Others will surely come after me, and perhaps I've given them something useful to mull over.

My family deserve the most acknowledgment. Thank you, Mom and Dad, for your unconditional love and tireless support. My older brother, Jim, appears in this book, and I commend his bravery and openness. Other family, like Ryan, Alison, Noah, and Ben, as well as Danette and Jeff McGilvray and the late Myrtle Munk, have been an important source of love and encouragement. My children, Aidric, Michaela, and Zora, appear now and then in the book, their stories thus far entangled with mine, and I hope someday they'll find something in here that they treasure. My most sincere gratitude goes to Tiffani Taggart, simultaneously stalwart, caring, and resilient, for putting up with me, for sharing her life with me—I cherish our journey so far with deep affection and admiration. None of this would be possible without her.

And again Michaela, of course, to whom this book is truly dedicated. It is my story, but the book is because of her.

Notes

CHAPTER 1. BECOMING

1. Peter Mandler, *Return from the Natives: How Margaret Mead Won the Second World War and Lost the Cold War* (New Haven, CT: Yale University Press, 2013).

2. Paul Austin, *Beautiful Eyes: A Father Transformed* (New York: W. W. Norton, 2014), 77.

3. Mandler, *Return from the Natives*, 26.

4. Lawrence Jacob Friedman, *Identity's Architect: A Biography of Erik H. Erikson* (Cambridge, MA: Harvard University Press, 2000), 209.

5. Charles King, *Gods of the Upper Air: How a Circle of Renegade Anthropologists Reinvented Race, Sex, and Gender in the Twentieth Century* (New York: Anchor Books, 2019).

6. *The Common Sense Book of Baby and Child Care* was published by Benjamin Spock in 1946, a now-famous guide that encourages parents to trust their judgement rather than follow overbearing rules or societal expectations.

7. Friedman, *Identity's Architect*, 209; Sue Erikson Bloland, *In the Shadow of Fame: A Memoir by the Daughter of Erik H. Erikson* (New York: Viking, 2006), 21; Roy Richard Grinker, *Nobody's Normal: How Culture Created the Stigma of Mental Illness* (New York: W. W. Norton, 2021), 195.

8. Bloland, *In the Shadow of Fame*, 24.

9. Incidence rates of Down syndrome worldwide are often estimated at around one out of every one thousand live births. The United States has a much

lower infant mortality rate than the worldwide average, which helps explain the difference. For specifics on Down syndrome in the United States, see "Data and Statistics on Down Syndrome," National Center on Birth Defects and Developmental Disabilities, Centers for Disease Control and Prevention, December 4, 2019, https://www.cdc.gov/ncbddd/birthdefects/downsyndrome/data.html.

10. Austin, *Beautiful Eyes*, 12.

11. Rayna Rapp, *Testing Women, Testing the Fetus: The Social Impact of Amniocentesis in America* (New York: Routledge, 2000), 271.

12. Chris Kaposy, *Choosing Down Syndrome: Ethics and New Prenatal Testing Technologies* (Cambridge, MA: MIT Press, 2018), 39.

13. King, *Gods of the Upper Air*.

14. In his book on the lives of fathers caring for their disabled children, the anthropologist Aaron Jackson describes "profound moments of disruption that move parents toward experiential disequilibrium. For many parents, their experience of a ruptured world lifts the veil on what was thought to be familiar and determinable, throwing light on taken-for-granted assumptions and the habits and routines of day-to-day life. A sense of continuity and predictability are displaced by a perceived mismatch between the present and a past that was supposed to lead somewhere else." See Aaron J. Jackson, *Worlds of Care: The Emotional Lives of Fathers Caring for Children with Disabilities* (Oakland: University of California Press, 2021), 31–32.

CHAPTER 2. FEATURES

1. John Langdon H. Down, "Observations on an Ethnic Classification of Idiots," *London Hospital Reports* 3 (1866): 259–62.

2. Stephen Jay Gould, *The Mismeasure of Man* (New York: W. W. Norton, 1996), 69.

3. Charles King, *Gods of the Upper Air: How a Circle of Renegade Anthropologists Reinvented Race, Sex, and Gender in the Twentieth Century* (New York: Anchor Books, 2019), 80.

4. Steven A. Gelb, "Darwin's Use of Intellectual Disability in The Descent of Man," *Disability Studies Quarterly* 28, no. 2 (2008), https://doi.org/10.18061/dsq.v28i2.96.

5. Gould, *Mismeasure of Man*, 74–82.

6. Gould, 114–39.

7. Kim E. Nielsen, *A Disability History of the United States* (Boston: Beacon Press, 2012), 57.

8. Nielsen, *Disability History*, 50.

9. Down, "Observations on an Ethnic Classification of Idiots."

10. David Wright, *Downs: The History of a Disability* (New York: Oxford University Press, 2011).

11. "From J. L. H. Down to Charles Darwin," December 18, 1873, Darwin Correspondence Project, https://www.darwinproject.ac.uk/letter/?docId=letters/DCP-LETT-9191.xml; "From J. L. H. Down to Charles Darwin," December 20, 1873, https://www.darwinproject.ac.uk/letter/DCP-LETT-9188.xml.

12. Gould, *Mismeasure of Man,* 143.

13. E. Peter Volpe, "Is Down Syndrome a Modern Disease?," *Perspectives in Biology and Medicine* 29, no. 3-1 (1986): 432.

14. Gelb, "Darwin's Use of Intellectual Disability in The Descent of Man."

15. Gould, *Mismeasure of Man,* 144.

16. Gould, 151–65.

17. Down, "Observations on an Ethnic Classification of Idiots."

18. Gould, *Mismeasure of Man,* 165.

19. Sunaura Taylor, *Beasts of Burden: Animal and Disability Liberation* (New York: New Press, 2017).

20. "From J. L. H. Down to Charles Darwin," December 20, 1873.

21. David Wright, "Mongols in Our Midst: John Langdon Down and the Ethnic Classification of Idiocy, 1858–1924," in *Mental Retardation in America: A Historical Reader,* ed. Steven Noll and James W. Trent (New York: New York University Press, 2004), 110.

22. Wright, "Mongols in Our Midst"; Wright, *Downs,* 48–80.

23. Nielsen, *Disability History,* 67.

24. Francis Galton, *Inquiries into Human Faculty and Its Development* (London: Macmillan, 1883), 24–25.

25. Disability studies scholars have argued that disability does not just intersect with or overlap with other differences such as race or gender, but rather that notions of racial difference are historically constituted through ideas about disability. See Nirmala Erevelles and Andrea Minear, "Unspeakable Offenses: Untangling Race and Disability in Discourses of Intersectionality," *Journal of Literacy and Cultural Disability Studies* 4, no. 2 (2010): 127–45.

26. Gould, *Mismeasure of Man,* 107.

27. Lennard J. Davis, "Introduction: Disability, Normality, and Power," in *The Disability Studies Reader,* ed. Lennard J. Davis, 5th ed. (New York: Routledge, 2017), 3.

28. Davis, "Introduction," 6.

29. James W. Trent, *Inventing the Feeble Mind: A History of Mental Retardation in the United States* (Berkeley: University of California Press, 1994), 140.

30. Gould, *Mismeasure of Man,* 178–84.

31. Gould, 187–88.

32. Gould, 189.

33. Gould, 199.

34. Henry Herbert Goddard, *The Kallikak Family: A Study in the Heredity of Feeblemindedness* (New York: Macmillan, 1921).

35. King, *Gods of the Upper Air*, 173–74.

36. Gould, *Mismeasure of Man*, 196.

37. Wright, *Downs*, 112–13.

38. Wright, 95.

39. Gould, *Mismeasure of Man*, 222.

40. Madison Grant, *The Passing of the Great Race: Or, The Racial Basis of European History* (New York: Charles Scribner's Sons, 1918).

41. Quoted in King, *Gods of the Upper Air*, 91.

42. Lee D. Baker, *From Savage to Negro: Anthropology and the Construction of Race, 1896–1954* (Berkeley: University of California Press, 1998).

43. Franz Boas, "Inventing a Great Race," *New Republic*, January 13, 1917. Also quoted in King, *Gods of the Upper Air*, 111.

44. King, *Gods of the Upper Air*, 121.

45. Ruth Benedict, "Anthropology and the Abnormal," *Journal of General Psychology* 10, no. 1 (1934): 73.

46. Wright, *Downs*, 80. Wright describes this as "a likelihood so improbable that it is scarcely believable, save for the lack of any historical evidence to suggest that the boy was, for example, an adopted patient of the institution."

47. O Conor Ward, "John Langdon Down: The Man and the Message," *Down Syndrome Research and Practice* 6, no. 1 (1999): 22. The photograph with Jonathan is reproduced in Wright, *Downs*, 75.

48. Deborah Cohen, *Family Secrets: Shame and Privacy in Modern Britain* (Oxford University Press, 2013), 101.

49. Cohen, *Family Secrets*, 101–2.

50. Wright, *Downs*, 82.

51. Cohen, *Family Secrets*, 99–101.

52. Wright, *Downs*, 114.

53. Quoted in Ward, "John Langdon Down," 21.

54. Francis Graham Crookshank, *The Mongol in Our Midst: A Study of Man and His Three Faces* (New York: E. P. Dutton, 1924), 21.

55. Michael Keevak, *Becoming Yellow: A Short History of Racial Thinking* (Princeton, NJ: Princeton University Press, 2011), 90–92.

56. Edward Sapir, "The Race Problem," *The Nation*, July 1, 1925.

57. Sapir, "Race Problem," 41.

58. Sapir, 41.

59. Francine Uenuma, "'Better Babies' Contests Pushed for Much-Needed Infant Health but Also Played into the Eugenics Movement," *Smithsonian Magazine*, January 17, 2019, https://www.smithsonianmag.com/history/better-babies-contests-pushed-infant-health-also-played-eugenics-movement-180971288/.

60. George Estreich, *Fables and Futures: Biotechnology, Disability, and the Stories We Tell Ourselves* (Cambridge, MA: MIT Press, 2019), 33.

61. Lee D. Baker, "The Racist Anti-Racism of American Anthropology," *Transforming Anthropology* 290, no. 2 (2020): 127–42; Audra Simpson, "Why White People Love Franz Boas; or, The Grammar of Indigenous Dispossession," in *Indigenous Visions: Rediscovering the World of Franz Boas,* ed. Ned Blackhawk and Isaiah Lorado Wilner, 166–81 (New Haven, CT: Yale University Press, 2018).

62. Margaret Mead, *Coming of Age in Samoa,* Laurel ed. (New York: Dell Publishing Company, [1928] 1968), 201.

63. There is an "absent presence" of disability in the ethnographic work of Boas and his students, in which various physical and cognitive conditions are noted in passing but never the focus of analysis. See Joshua Reno et al., "Toward a Critical and Comparative Anthropology of Disability: Absent Presence and Exemplary Personhood," *Social Analysis* 65, no. 3 (September 1, 2021): 131–49, https://doi.org/10.3167/sa.2021.650307.

CHAPTER 3. INSTITUTIONS

1. Michael J. Goc, ed., *Island of Refuge: The Northern Wisconsin Center for the Developmentally Disabled, 1897–1997* (Friendship, WI: New Past Press, 1997), 12.

2. Charles is described in Goc, *Island of Refuge,* a centennial self-history of the institution, as the architect contracted to design the Home for the Feebleminded in 1896, including the administration building, and his name appears in historical documents associated with the home. Originally based out of Menomonie, he was commissioned by the State Board of Control to design other public buildings and moved his offices to Madison. The Wisconsin Historical Society credits him with the design of many buildings at the Wisconsin Home for the Feebleminded, but curiously lists Van Ryn and De Gelleke as the architects for the administration building. Construction of buildings at the Home for the Feeble-Minded occurred regularly until 1915.

3. Goc, *Island of Refuge.*

4. Ed Treleven, "State Settles Lawsuit over Center Closing," *Chippewa Herald,* August 3, 2004, https://chippewa.com/news/state-settles-lawsuit-over-center-closing/article_aeb66667-74d9-5c0e-8c29-adf1a5309140.html.

5. A. W. Wilmarth, "Heredity as a Social Burden," *Journal of the American Medical Association* 27, no. 7 (1896): 341–44.

6. David Wright, *Downs: The History of a Disability* (New York: Oxford University Press, 2011), 70.

7. Goc, *Island of Refuge,* 18.

8. Goc, 28.

9. In "The Operation and Administration of the Northern Wisconsin Colony and Training School," published in 1938, Irene Beier wrote: "In a feeble-minded person the animal passions are usually present and are often abnormally developed. The feeble-minded woman is perhaps the worst offender. She cannot resist the persuasions and temptations that beset her. Society needs to be protected from her. . . . Irresponsible and innocent of intentional wrong, she brings to our very doors the most destructive and insidious of evils." Irene Beier was the daughter of Augustus L. Beier, assistant superintendent of the Wisconsin Home from 1908 to 1919, and superintendent from 1919 until 1940. Irene Beier is quoted in Anna G. Mirer, "Wisconsin's Strange History of State-Sponsored Sterilization," *Worse for the Fishes: A Safety Valve for the Opinions of Anna G. Mirer, Ph.D., M.P.H* (blog), August 21, 2016, https://annamirer.wordpress.com/2016/08/21/wisconsins-strange-history-of-state-sponsored-sterilization/.

10. A. W. Wilmarth, "Superintendent's Report," *Fifth Biennial Report of the Home for the Feeble-Minded, for the Biennial Period Ending June 30, 1906* (Madison: Democrat Printing, 1906), available at https://hdl.handle.net/2027/wu.89102772480.

11. James W. Trent, *Inventing the Feeble Mind: A History of Mental Retardation in the United States* (Berkeley: University of California Press, 1994).

12. Adam Seth Cohen, *Imbeciles: The Supreme Court, American Eugenics, and the Sterilization of Carrie Buck* (New York: Penguin Press, 2016), 24.

13. Mark G. Bold, "Op-Ed: It's Time for California to Compensate Its Forced-Sterilization Victims," *Los Angeles Times,* March 5, 2015, https://www.latimes.com/opinion/op-ed/la-oe-0306-bold-forced-sterilization-compensation-20150306-story.html.

14. Wright, *Downs,* 103–8.

15. Scott Gordon, "The Painful History of Eugenics in Wisconsin," *WisContext,* October 6, 2016, https://www.wiscontext.org/painful-history-eugenics-wisconsin.

16. Phyllis E. Reske, "Policing the 'Wayward Woman': Eugenics in Wisconsin's Involuntary Sterilization Program," *Wisconsin Magazine of History,* Autumn 2013.

17. Goc, *Island of Refuge,* 155.

18. John Brassard Jr., "Deadly Delivery," *The Kitchen Table Historian* (blog), May 29, 2019, https://johnbrassardjr.com/2019/05/29/deadly-delivery/.

19. Goc, *Island of Refuge,* 155.

20. A. W. Wilmarth, "Superintendent's Report," *Tenth Biennial Report of the Wisconsin Home for the Feeble-Minded, Located at Chippewa Falls, for the Biennial Period Ending June 30, 1916* (Madison: State Board of Control of Wisconsin, 1916), https://hdl.handle.net/2027/wu.89102772548.

21. Thomas C. Leonard, *Illiberal Reformers: Race, Eugenics, and American Economics in the Progressive Era* (Princeton, NJ: Princeton University Press, 2016).

22. Jonathan Peter Spiro, *Defending the Master Race: Conservation, Eugenics, and the Legacy of Madison Grant* (Lebanon, NH: University Press of New England, 2009), 137.

23. "Subject Syllabi in Home and Social Economics, 1913–14: Eugenics," Stout Small Series 2, vol. 3, The Stout Institute, July 1913, University Archives and Area Research Center, University of Wisconsin-Stout.

24. Two historic late nineteenth-century buildings at the center of the UW-Stout campus demonstrate this: As originally designed, Harvey Hall was accessible only through exterior and interior staircases leading to a grand lobby, and millions of dollars have been spent to retrofit the building. Bowman Hall was also once accessible only by staircase, but the exterior staircase was removed, and landscaping regraded to make it accessible at some point in the 1980s.

25. Jay T. Dolmage, *Academic Ableism: Disability and Higher Education* (Ann Arbor: University of Michigan Press, 2017).

26. Carla Yanni, *The Architecture of Madness: Insane Asylums in the United States* (Minneapolis: University of Minnesota Press, 2007).

27. Mirer, "Wisconsin's Strange History of State-Sponsored Sterilization."

28. Goc, *Island of Refuge*, 40.

29. Gordon, "The Painful History of Eugenics in Wisconsin."

30. One publication from that research was in *American Anthropologist*, which became the flagship journal of the American Anthropological Association (AAA). Originally founded in 1888, the journal was relaunched in 1899 with an editorial board that included Franz Boas. The AAA was established in 1902, and Franz Boas (1907–8), Edward Sapir (1938), Ruth Benedict (1947), and Margaret Mead (1960) each served as its president.

31. Roy Richard Grinker, *Nobody's Normal: How Culture Created the Stigma of Mental Illness* (New York: W. W. Norton, 2021), xxiii.

32. Grinker, *Nobody's Normal*.

CHAPTER 4. POTENTIAL

1. *Margaret Mead: An Observer Observed*, directed by Alan Berliner (New York: Filmakers Library, 1996).

2. Patrick McKearney and Tyler Zoanni, "Introduction: For an Anthropology of Cognitive Disability," *Cambridge Journal of Anthropology* 36, no. 1 (2018): 4.

3. Recent work by anthropologists on autism, and on how caregivers relate to severely disabled children amid the absence of language, has more deeply explored how people with cognitive disabilities relate to both language and the social world differently. See, for instance, Roy Richard Grinker, *Unstrange Minds: Remapping the World of Autism* (New York: Basic Books, 2007); Aaron J. Jackson, *Worlds of Care: The Emotional Lives of Fathers Caring for Children*

with Disabilities (Oakland: University of California Press, 2021); Elinor Ochs and Olga Solomon, "Autistic Sociality," *Ethos* 38, no. 1 (2010): 69–92.

4. Rayna Rapp, *Testing Women, Testing the Fetus: The Social Impact of Amniocentesis in America* (New York: Routledge, 2000), 273.

5. Paul Shankman, "The Public Anthropology of Margaret Mead: *Redbook*, Women's Issues, and the 1960s," *Current Anthropology* 59, no. 1 (2018): 55–73.

6. Shankman, "Public Anthropology of Margaret Mead," 57.

7. Margaret Mead, "Margaret Mead Answers: What Is the Modern Grandparent's Role? What Happens to Exceptional Children in Primitive Societies? Has the Medicine Man Anything in Common with the Psychoanalyst?," *Redbook*, June 1966, 30.

8. Glen Doss, "The Controversial Margaret Mead," *Stars and Stripes*, June 2, 1972, https://www.stripes.com/news/the-controversial-margaret-mead-1.14098.

9. Joel Goldberg, "It Takes a Village to Determine the Origins of an African Proverb," *Goats and Soda: Stories of Life in a Changing World*, July 30, 2016, https://www.npr.org/sections/goatsandsoda/2016/07/30/487925796/it-takes-a-village-to-determine-the-origins-of-an-african-proverb.

10. Margaret Mead, "Can the American Family Survive?," *Redbook*, February 1977, 161.

11. "The Cost of Child Care in Wisconsin," Economic Policy Institute, accessed June 18, 2021, https://www.epi.org/child-care-costs-in-the-united-states/.

12. Lawrence Jacob Friedman, *Identity's Architect: A Biography of Erik H. Erikson* (Cambridge, MA: Harvard University Press, 2000), 209.

13. Allison C. Carey, *On the Margins of Citizenship: Intellectual Disability and Civil Rights in Twentieth-Century America* (Philadelphia: Temple University Press, 2010), 90.

14. Carey, *On the Margins of Citizenship*, 90.

15. Shankman, "Public Anthropology of Margaret Mead," 63.

16. Carey, *On the Margins of Citizenship*, 105.

17. Carey, 106.

18. Carey, 107–8.

19. Pearl S. Buck, "The Child Who Never Grew," *Ladies' Home Journal*, May 1950, 34–35, 146–50, 152, 154, 156, 159–60, 163, 165, 167, 169.

20. Carey, *On the Margins of Citizenship*, 110.

21. Buck, "The Child Who Never Grew," 159.

22. Quoted in Carey, *On the Margins of Citizenship*, 110.

23. Buck, "The Child Who Never Grew," 169; also quoted in Carey, *On the Margins of Citizenship*, 111.

24. Carey, *On the Margins of Citizenship*, 111–12.

25. Carey, 112.

26. Eva Feder Kittay, "Forever Small: The Strange Case of Ashley X," *Hypatia* 26, no. 3 (2011): 610–31, https://doi.org/10.1111/j.1527-2001.2011.01205.x.

27. Buck, "The Child Who Never Grew," 152.

28. "Pity Is Deplored for the Handicapped: Anthropologist Says 'Triumph Over Circumstances' Ought to Be Element Stressed," *New York Times*, November 6, 1954.

29. "A Conversation with Margaret Mead and William Mitchell," *Wisdom*, aired 1959, NBC.

30. Shankman, "Public Anthropology of Margaret Mead," 56.

31. Wolf Wolfensberger, "The Fiftieth Anniversary of What Appears to Be the World's First Doctoral Degree Program in Mental Retardation: Some Reminiscences of an Early Graduate," *Intellectual and Developmental Disabilities* 46, no. 1 (2008): 73.

32. Carey, *On the Margins of Citizenship*, 97–98.

33. Council on Developmental Disabilities, "The Parent Groups and Professional Organizations," Parallels in Time: A History of Developmental Disabilities, MN Department of Administration, accessed January 20, 2021, https://mn.gov/mnddc/parallels/five/5a/3.html.

34. Terrell Harris Dougan, *That Went Well: Adventures in Caring for My Sister* (New York: Hachette Books, 2009).

35. Council on Developmental Disabilities, "Improve the Institutions," Parallels in Time: A History of Developmental Disabilities, MN Department of Administration, accessed January 20, 2021, https://mn.gov/mnddc/parallels/five/5a/11.html.

36. Quoted in Carey, *On the Margins of Citizenship*, 101.

37. Wolfensberger, "Fiftieth Anniversary," 73.

38. An edited transcript of her remarks was prepared as part of the symposium proceedings and published in the AAMD's journal. See Margaret Mead, "Research: Cult or Cure?," *American Journal of Mental Deficiency* 64 (1959): 253–64.

39. Seymour B. Sarason and Thomas Gladwin, "Psychological and Cultural Problems in Mental Subnormality," *Genetic Psychology Monographs* 57 (1958): 3–289; Richard L. Masland, Seymour B. Sarason, and Thomas Gladwin, *Mental Subnormality: Biological, Psychological, and Cultural Factors* (New York: Basic Books, 1958).

40. Even the tenth edition, edited in 1963 by Roger Francis Tredgold and Kenneth Soddy, and published as "Tredgold's Textbook of Mental Deficiency (Subnormality)," stated that "man, having once begun to interfere with nature [through selective breeding], must go on with the job if he would escape wreckage and social catastrophe. The question is, how? The drastic proposal of euthanasia has been made, and must be considered." Alfred Frank Tredgold, Roger Francis Tredgold, and Kenneth Soddy, *Textbook of Mental Deficiency (Subnormality)*

(Baltimore: Williams and Wilkins Co., 1963), 469–70, available at http://archive
.org/details/textbookofmentae10tred.

41. Wolfensberger, "Fiftieth Anniversary," 70.

42. Mead, "Research: Cult or Cure?," 253.

43. Masland, Sarason, and Gladwin, *Mental Subnormality,* 145.

44. Marvin K. Opler, "Review of 'Mental Subnormality: Biological, Psychological and Cultural Factors,' by Richard L. Masland, Seymour B. Sarason, and Thomas Gladwin," *American Anthropologist* 61, no. 6 (1959): 1161.

45. Weston La Barre, "Review of 'Psychological and Cultural Problems in Mental Subnormality: A Review of Research,' by Seymour B. Sarason and Thomas Gladwin," *American Anthropologist* 61, no. 1 (1959): 166–67.

46. Mead, "Research: Cult or Cure?," 255–56.

47. Mead, 256.

48. Albert Q. Maisel, "Bedlam 1946," *Life,* May 6, 1946, 103.

49. Carey, *On the Margins of Citizenship,* 92.

50. Carey, 85; James W. Trent, *Inventing the Feeble Mind: A History of Mental Retardation in the United States* (Berkeley: University of California Press, 1994), 240.

51. Burton Blatt and Fred Kaplan, *Christmas in Purgatory: A Photographic Essay on Mental Retardation* (Syracuse, NY: Human Policy Press, 1974), v.

52. Blatt and Kaplan, *Christmas in Purgatory,* 34.

53. Carey, *On the Margins of Citizenship,* 92.

54. Erving Goffman, "Interpersonal Persuasion," in *Group Processes: Transactions of the Third Conference,* ed. Bertram Schaffner, 117–93 (New York: Madison Printing Company, 1957).

55. Mead, "Research: Cult or Cure?," 257.

56. Mead, 258.

57. Mead, 259.

58. Mead, 260.

59. Mead, 261.

60. Mead, 262.

61. Allison C. Carey, Pamela Block, and Richard Scotch, *Allies and Obstacles: Disability Activism and Parents of Children with Disabilities* (Philadelphia: Temple University Press, 2020).

62. Evelyn West Ayrault, *You Can Raise Your Handicapped Child* (New York: G. P. Putnam's Sons, 1964), 15.

63. Carey, *On the Margins of Citizenship,* 95.

64. Kim E. Nielsen, *A Disability History of the United States* (Boston: Beacon Press, 2012), 150–55.

65. Margaret Mead, "Dr. Margaret Mead's Address," in *Annual Meeting Minutes: The President's Committee on Employment of the Handicapped* (Washington, DC: Bureau of Labor Standards, 1967), 7.

66. Mead, "Dr. Margaret Mead's Address," 8.

67. Mead, 8.

68. Mead, 9.

69. "Papua New Guinea: Sex and Temperament," Margaret Mead: Human Nature and the Power of Culture, Library of Congress, November 30, 2001, https://www.loc.gov/exhibits/mead/field-sepik.html.

70. Mead, "Dr. Margaret Mead's Address," 9.

71. John Langston Gwaltney, "Some Thoughts on Native Anthropology," *Transforming Anthropology* 7, no. 2 (1998): 67–69.

72. Lesley A. Sharp, "The Ethnographic Vision of John L. Gwaltney: *The Thrice Shy*, a Forgotten Gem," *Somatosphere*, July 24, 2015, http://somatosphere.net/2015/the-ethnographic-vision-of-john-l-gwaltney-the-thrice-shy-a-forgotten-gem.html/.

73. John Langston Gwaltney, *The Thrice Shy: Cultural Accommodation to Blindness and Other Disasters in a Mexican Community* (New York: Columbia University Press, 1970).

74. Sharp, "The Ethnographic Vision of John L. Gwaltney."

75. Gwaltney, *The Thrice Shy*, 1–2.

76. John Langston Gwaltney, "The Blind of San Pedro Yolox," *American Scholar* 35, no. 1 (1965): 116–17.

77. Gwaltney, "The Blind of San Pedro Yolox," 117.

78. Sharp, "The Ethnographic Vision of John L. Gwaltney."

79. Gwaltney, "The Blind of San Pedro Yolox," 125.

80. Mead, "Dr. Margaret Mead's Address," 8.

81. Margaret Mead, "A Mother's Day Message: What We Can Do Now for Our Children's Future," *Redbook*, May 1979, 198.

82. Eunice Kennedy Shriver, "Hope for Retarded Children," *Saturday Evening Post*, September 22, 1962, 72.

83. Carey, *On the Margins of Citizenship*, 127–28.

84. Margaret Mead, "Statement of Dr. Margaret Mead to the 1969 Joint Commission on Mental Health of Children," in *Departments of Labor, Health and Human Services, Education, and Related Agencies Appropriations for 1984; Hearings Before a Subcommittee of the Committee on Appropriations, House of Representatives, Ninety-Eighth Congress, First Session; Part 8, Testimony of Members of Congress and Interested Individuals and Organizations* (Washington, DC: U.S. Government Printing Office, 1983), 675.

85. Carey, *On the Margins of Citizenship*, 140–41.

86. Carey, 141.

87. Wolf Wolfensberger, *The Principle of Normalization in Human Services* (Toronto: National Institute on Mental Retardation, 1972).

88. Carey, *On the Margins of Citizenship*, 147.

89. Mead, "Mother's Day Message," 196, 198.

90. Lennard J. Davis, *Enabling Acts: The Hidden Story of How the Americans with Disability Act Gave the Largest U.S. Minority Its Rights* (Boston: Beacon Press, 2016).

91. Carey, *On the Margins of Citizenship*, 205.

92. This reflects the shifting, situational meanings associated with disability categories and terms. Other scholars have written about the alienation that parents often endure when, in order to access services for their children, they are obligated to participate in pathologizing ways of thinking and to utilize medicalized categories that rarely reflect how they perceive their children. Jackson notes that parents are often "deeply aware of the practices that diminish the humanity of children with disabilities. A problem parents face, then, is how to go about transcending these painful situations and carving out spaces of belonging where their children might be experienced otherwise." Jackson, *Worlds of Care*, 124; see also Faye Ginsburg and Rayna Rapp, "Entangled Ethnography: Imagining a Future for Young Adults with Learning Disabilities," *Social Science and Medicine* 99 (December 2013): 187–93, https://doi.org/10.1016/j.socscimed.2013.11.015; Tom Shakespeare, *Disability: The Basics* (New York: Routledge, 2018), 52.

CHAPTER 5. BELONGING

1. Alison Piepmeier, *Unexpected: Parenting, Prenatal Testing, and Down Syndrome*, with George Estreich and Rachel Adams (New York: NYU Press, 2021), 27.

2. For an insightful discussion of elopement (or bolting), and strategies to manage that behavior, see David S. Stein, *Supporting Positive Behavior in Children and Teens with Down Syndrome: The Respond but Don't React Method* (Bethesda, MD: Woodbine House, 2016).

3. Fiona Kumari Campbell, *Contours of Ableism: The Production of Disability and Abledness* (New York: Palgrave Macmillan, 2009), 17; for an insightful discussion of ableism, see also Sunaura Taylor, *Beasts of Burden: Animal and Disability Liberation* (New York: New Press, 2017), 3–21.

4. See Aaron J. Jackson, *Worlds of Care: The Emotional Lives of Fathers Caring for Children with Disabilities* (Oakland: University of California Press, 2021), 130–32; see also Rosemarie Garland-Thomson, *Staring: How We Look* (New York: Oxford University Press, 2009).

5. Lawrence Jacob Friedman, *Identity's Architect: A Biography of Erik H. Erikson* (Cambridge, MA: Harvard University Press, 2000), 210.

6. Friedman, *Identity's Architect*, 210.

7. Friedman, 211; Sue Erikson Bloland, *In the Shadow of Fame: A Memoir by the Daughter of Erik H. Erikson* (New York: Viking, 2006), 36.

8. Friedman, *Identity's Architect*, 213.

9. Friedman, 213.

10. Friedman, 213–14.

11. Bloland, *In the Shadow of Fame*, 25.

12. Bloland, 91.

13. Bloland, 104.

14. Friedman, *Identity's Architect*, 214.

15. Bloland, *In the Shadow of Fame*, 109.

16. Bloland, 109–10.

17. David Wright, *Downs: The History of a Disability* (New York: Oxford University Press, 2011), 122.

18. Gordon Allen et al., "Mongolism," *The Lancet* 277, no. 7180 (April 8, 1961): 775. The letter was republished the same year in the *American Journal of Human Genetics*. See Gordon Allen et al., "Mongolism," *American Journal of Human Genetics* 13, no. 4 (December 1961): 426.

19. Kristin Kelley, "Amniocentesis Prior to 1980," *Embryo Project Encyclopedia*, September 2, 2010, https://embryo.asu.edu/handle/10776/2072.

20. George Estreich, *Fables and Futures: Biotechnology, Disability, and the Stories We Tell Ourselves* (Cambridge, MA: MIT Press, 2019), 132.

21. Bernard Bard and Joseph Fletcher, "The Right to Die," *Atlantic Monthly*, April 1968, 59–64.

22. Bard and Fletcher, "The Right to Die," 64.

23. Jacqueline A. Noonan, "A History of Pediatric Specialties: The Development of Pediatric Cardiology," *Pediatric Research* 56, no. 2 (August 2004): 298–306, https://doi.org/10.1203/01.PDR.0000132662.73362.96.

24. Norman Fost, "'The Hopkins Mongol Case': The Dawn of the Bioethics Movement," *Pediatrics* 146, no. s1 (2020): 5.

25. George J. Annas, "Denying the Rights of the Retarded: The Phillip Becker Case," *Hastings Center Report* 9, no. 6 (1979): 18, https://doi.org/10.2307/3561672.

26. Fost, "The Hopkins Mongol Case."

27. Annas, "Denying the Rights of the Retarded."

28. Fost, "The Hopkins Mongol Case," 5.

29. Michael White, "The End at the Beginning," *Ochsner Journal* 11, no. 4 (2011): 309–16.

30. Emily Rapp, *The Still Point of the Turning World* (New York: Penguin, 2014).

31. Fost, "The Hopkins Mongol Case."

32. Andrew Solomon, *Far from the Tree: Parents, Children, and the Search for Identity* (New York: Simon and Schuster, 2012), 171–79.

33. Joan Ganz Cooney, "Foreword," in *Count Us In: Growing Up with Down Syndrome* (Orlando, FL: Mariner Books, 2007), viii–x.

34. Michael Bérubé, *Life as We Know It: A Father, a Family, and an Exceptional Child* (New York: Vintage Books, 1998), 6.

35. Rayna Rapp, *Testing Women, Testing the Fetus: The Social Impact of Amniocentesis in America* (New York: Routledge, 2000), 290.

36. See also, for instance: Rachel Adams, *Raising Henry: A Memoir of Motherhood, Disability, and Discovery* (New Haven, CT: Yale University Press, 2013); Paul Austin, *Beautiful Eyes: A Father Transformed* (New York: W. W. Norton, 2014); Michael Bérubé, *Life as Jamie Knows It: An Exceptional Child Grows Up* (Boston: Beacon Press, 2016); Victoria Freeman, *A World without Martha: A Memoir of Sisters, Disability, and Difference* (Vancouver: University of British Columbia Press, 2019); George Estreich, *The Shape of the Eye: A Memoir* (New York: Penguin, 2013); Piepmeier, *Unexpected.*

37. Helga Kuhse and Peter Singer, *Should the Baby Live? The Problem of Handicapped Infants* (New York: Oxford University Press, 1985); Peter Singer, *Rethinking Life and Death: The Collapse of Our Traditional Ethics* (New York: St. Martin's Griffin, 1994).

38. Singer, *Rethinking Life and Death*, 213; also quoted in Michael Bérubé, "Equality, Freedom, and/or Justice for All: A Response to Martha Nussbaum," *Metaphilosophy* 40, no. 3/4 (2009): 353.

39. For criticism of his views, see Harriet McBryde Johnson, "Unspeakable Conversations," *New York Times Magazine*, February 16, 2003, https://www.nytimes.com/2003/02/16/magazine/unspeakable-conversations.html; Tom Shakespeare, *Disability: The Basics* (New York: Routledge, 2018), 122; Bérubé, *Life as Jamie Knows It*; Taylor, *Beasts of Burden.*

40. Rayna Rapp, "The Ethics of Choice," *Ms.*, April 1984, 97.

41. Rapp, "Ethics of Choice," 97.

42. Rapp, 98.

43. Rapp, 99.

44. Rapp, 98.

45. Rapp, *Testing Women, Testing the Fetus*, 17.

46. Rapp, *Testing Women, Testing the Fetus*, 106; see also Gail Landsman, *Reconstructing Motherhood and Disability in the Age of Perfect Babies* (New York: Routledge, 2008).

47. Gareth M. Thomas, *Down's Syndrome Screening and Reproductive Politics: Care, Choice, and Disability in the Prenatal Clinic* (New York: Routledge, 2017), 160–67.

48. Rapp, *Testing Women, Testing the Fetus*, 131.

49. Rayna Rapp, "After Mead," in "Margaret Mead's Legacy: Continuing Conversations," special issue, *Scholar and Feminist Online* 1, no. 2 (2003), http://sfonline.barnard.edu/mead/rapp.htm. See also Esther Newton, *Margaret Mead Made Me Gay: Personal Essays, Public Ideas* (Durham, NC: Duke University Press, 2000).

50. Faye D. Ginsburg and Rayna Rapp, eds., *Conceiving the New World Order: The Global Politics of Reproduction* (Berkeley: University of California Press, 1995).

51. Following her work on the social impacts of amniocentesis, Rapp, along with her collaborator Faye Ginsburg, would become a pivotal figure in anthropology's growing engagement with disability studies and the project of understanding disability as difference. See, for instance, Rayna Rapp and Faye Ginsburg, "Reverberations: Disability and the New Kinship Imaginary," *Anthropological Quarterly* 84, no. 2 (2011): 379–410; Faye Ginsburg and Rayna Rapp, "Disability Worlds," *Annual Review of Anthropology* 42 (2013): 53–68; Faye Ginsburg and Rayna Rapp, "Disability/Anthropology: Rethinking the Parameters of the Human: An Introduction to Supplement 21," *Current Anthropology* 61, no. s21 (2020): s4–15; Faye Ginsburg and Rayna Rapp, "Cognitive Disability: Towards an Ethics of Possibility," *Cambridge Journal of Anthropology* 36, no. 1 (2018): 113–19.

52. Rapp, "Ethics of Choice," 99. She continues: "The disability rights movement has raised the question of eugenics, and the goal of making it 'cheaper' and 'more acceptable' to screen for genetically 'perfect' fetuses than to support the services disabled children need. While health economists may find amniocentesis and abortion more 'cost effective' than caring for special-needs children, as feminists we need to acknowledge that such lives are worth living. At the same time, we know that a woman needs access to abortion for whatever reasons she chooses not to bear a specific pregnancy to term. Our commitment to abortion goes hand in hand with an equally strong commitment to decent prenatal care, child care, education, and health services for children women do bear. The same connections must be made in support of disability rights. Any woman may decide she will not bear a specific fetus, once prenatal diagnosis reveals a serious disability she does not want to live with. But every feminist should support the rights . . . of the disabled."

53. The *New York Times* reported on a 2014 study which "found that 6 percent of patients who screened positive obtained an abortion without getting another test to confirm the result." Sarah Kliff and Aatish Bhatia, "When They Warn of Rare Disorders, These Prenatal Tests Are Usually Wrong," *New York Times,* January 1, 2022, https://www.nytimes.com/2022/01/01/upshot/pregnancy-birth-genetic-testing.html.

54. Estreich, *Fables and Futures,* xiv.

55. Michael Gerson, "The Eugenics Temptation," *Washington Post,* October 24, 2007, http://www.washingtonpost.com/wp-dyn/content/article/2007/10/23/AR2007102301803.html.

56. Estreich, *Fables and Futures,* 15.

57. Estreich, 17.

58. Jennifer A. Doudna and Samuel H. Sternberg, *A Crack in Creation: Gene Editing and the Unthinkable Power to Control Evolution* (Boston: Houghton Mifflin Harcourt, 2017), quoted in Estreich, 17.

59. "Early Risk Assessment of Down Syndrome and Other Conditions," MaterniT 21 PLUS Test, Labcorp, accessed October 14, 2021, https://www.integratedgenetics.com/patients/pregnancy/maternit21plus.

60. Estreich, *Fables and Futures*, 49.

61. A *New York Times* analysis found that companies increasingly promote NIPT for extremely rare conditions such as DiGeorge syndrome, 1p36 deletion, cri du chat syndrome, Wolf-Hirschhorn syndrome, Prader-Willi syndrome, and Angelman syndrome. For these conditions, the frequency of false positives range from 81 percent to 93 percent. See Kliff and Bhatia, "When They Warn of Rare Disorders."

62. Estreich, *Fables and Futures*, 56.

63. Chris Kaposy, *Choosing Down Syndrome: Ethics and New Prenatal Testing Technologies* (Cambridge, MA: MIT Press, 2018), 16.

64. Negative attitudes about disability are often grounded in assumptions about the future, imagined as difficult, as fraught with inevitable suffering, as characterized by burdens that must be overcome, or as hopeless. Rethinking disability in relation to how we conceive of difference and belonging entails imagining alternative futures as well as broader, more inclusive conceptions of humanity. See, for instance, Alison Kafer, *Feminist, Queer, Crip* (Bloomington: Indiana University Press, 2013); Rosemarie Garland-Thomson, "A Habitable World: Harriet McBryde Johnson's 'Case for My Life,'" *Hypatia* 30, no. 1 (2015): 300–306; Gareth Thomas, "Un/Inhabitable Worlds: The Curious Case of Down's Syndrome," *Somatosphere*, July 29, 2015, http://somatosphere.net/2015/uninhabitable-worlds-the-curious-case-of-downs-syndrome.html/; Faye Ginsburg and Rayna Rapp, "Entangled Ethnography: Imagining a Future for Young Adults with Learning Disabilities," *Social Science and Medicine* 99 (December 2013): 187–93, https://doi.org/10.1016/j.socscimed.2013.11.015.

65. Estreich, *Fables and Futures*, 49.

66. Kaposy, *Choosing Down Syndrome*, 4.

67. Sarah Zhang, "The Last Children of Down Syndrome," *The Atlantic*, December 2020, 44.

68. Erik Parens and Adrienne Asch, "The Disability Rights Critique of Prenatal Genetic Testing: Reflections and Recommendations," *Hastings Center Report* 29, no. 5 (1999): s1–22.

69. Thomas, *Down's Syndrome Screening and Reproductive Politics*, 134.

70. Rosemarie Garland-Thomson, "Human Biodiversity Conservation: A Consensual Ethical Principle," *American Journal of Bioethics* 15, no. 6 (June 2015): 14, https://doi.org/10.1080/15265161.2015.1028663.

71. Amy Julia Becker, "I'm Thankful Every Day for the Decision I Made after My Prenatal Tests," *New York Times*, February 1, 2022, https://www.nytimes.com/2022/02/01/opinion/prenatal-testing.html.

72. Estreich, *Fables and Futures*, xvi.

73. In a now famous essay, the philosopher Michael Sandel argues that society's investment in biomedical enhancement of the human condition has profound moral consequences, in the case of parenting, eroding the norms of

"unconditional love" and an "openness to the unbidden." We can never really predict or control how our kids' lives turn out; pretending this is possible has deep cultural implications. See Michael J. Sandel, *The Case against Perfection: Ethics in the Age of Genetic Engineering* (Cambridge, MA: Belknap Press, 2007).

74. Margaret Mead, *Culture and Commitment: A Study of the Generation Gap* (New York: Doubleday, 1970), 88–89.

CHAPTER 6. VULNERABILITY

1. Paul E. Farmer et al., "Structural Violence and Clinical Medicine," *PLOS Medicine* 3, no. 10 (October 24, 2006): 1686, https://doi.org/10.1371/journal.pmed.0030449. See also Paul Farmer, "On Suffering and Structural Violence: A View from Below," *Daedalus* 125, no. 1 (1996): 261–83; Paul Farmer, "An Anthropology of Structural Violence," *Current Anthropology* 45, no. 3 (2004): 305–25, https://doi.org/10.1086/382250.

2. Caitlin Dickerson and Miriam Jordan, "South Dakota Meat Plant Is Now Country's Biggest Coronavirus Hot Spot," *New York Times*, April 15, 2020, https://www.nytimes.com/2020/04/15/us/coronavirus-south-dakota-meat-plant-refugees.html.

3. By September 2020, at least four Smithfield plant workers had died from COVID-19, adding to the more than two hundred meat plant workers across the United States who lost their lives to the disease up to that point. See Kimberly Kindy, "More than 200 Meat Plant Workers in the U.S. Have Died of Covid-19. Federal Regulators Just Issued Two Modest Fines," *Washington Post*, September 13, 2020, https://www.washingtonpost.com/national/osha-covid-meat-plant-fines/2020/09/13/1dca3e14-f395-11ea-bc45-e5d48ab44b9f_story.html.

4. Daniel Wood, "As Pandemic Deaths Add Up, Racial Disparities Persist—and in Some Cases Worsen," *Shots: Health News from NPR*, September 23, 2020, https://www.npr.org/sections/health-shots/2020/09/23/914427907/as-pandemic-deaths-add-up-racial-disparities-persist-and-in-some-cases-worsen.

5. Several factors help explain such patterns, though it's important to acknowledge that any given place or community will be shaped by its unique historical context. In general, however, racial discrimination and class inequality play significant roles. Many American cities are shaped by a history of residential segregation rooted in early twentieth-century Jim Crow laws and institutional racism. The midcentury trend of suburban development was molded by discriminatory practices in real estate development and lending that predominately channeled availability of low-cost mortgages to White borrowers, setting into motion the reproduction of White generational wealth in the form of home ownership but also pushing people of color into less desirable urban and suburban enclaves. Poverty and social disadvantage are associated with higher incidences of

underlying health problems that are among the risk factors for severe COVID-19 disease, such as obesity, diabetes, high blood pressure, heart disease, and asthma. Many of these chronic health conditions are caused or exacerbated by the life circumstances in which inadequate nutrition, degraded air quality, stress, lack of free time for exercise, and subpar educational opportunities interact with human biology to generate negative health outcomes, to impair and disable people. As a result of urban and suburban residential segregation, racially marginalized groups are more likely to live or work in unhealthy neighborhoods located near industry or interstate highways that contribute to air pollution, serviced by old municipal water systems prone to deterioration and heighted risk of lead contamination, or to be dependent on jobs with increased risk of occupational health hazards. When dealing with illness, many people in the United States also encounter barriers to accessing healthcare treatment, or even basic precautionary measures such as COVID-19 testing, due to the country's fragmented healthcare system, gaps in insurance coverage, and costs associated with seeing a doctor. Once at the doctor's office, people of color are also more likely to be subject to unconscious bias in their treatment, encountering doctors or nurses who downplay or disregard their complaints of pain and discomfort, or prematurely release ailing patients. As a result of deeply rooted racial disparities in the criminal justice system, people of color are also dramatically overrepresented in jails, prisons, and detention centers. While during the first year of the pandemic the United States had the highest infection rate in the world, the rate of infection in U.S. prisons was three times higher than in the general population. For reporting on how these social and economic disparities informed the experience of COVID-19, see John Eligon et al., "Black Americans Face Alarming Rates of Coronavirus Infection in Some States," *New York Times*, April 7, 2020, https://www.nytimes.com/2020/04/07/us/coronavirus-race.html; Wood, "As Pandemic Deaths Add Up"; Linda Villarosa and L. Kasimu Harris, "'A Terrible Price': The Deadly Racial Disparities of Covid-19 in America," *New York Times Magazine*, April 29, 2020, https://www.nytimes.com/2020/04/29/magazine/racial-disparities-covid-19.html; Hiroko Tabuchi, "In the Shadows of America's Smokestacks, Virus Is One More Deadly Risk," *New York Times*, May 17, 2020, https://www.nytimes.com/2020/05/17/climate/pollution-poverty-coronavirus.html; John Eligon and Audra D. S. Burch, "Questions of Bias in Covid-19 Treatment Add to the Mourning for Black Families," *New York Times*, May 10, 2020, https://www.nytimes.com/2020/05/10/us/coronavirus-african-americans-bias.html; Eddie Burkhalter et al., "Incarcerated and Infected: How the Virus Tore through the U.S. Prison System," *New York Times*, April 10, 2021, https://www.nytimes.com/interactive/2021/04/10/us/covid-prison-outbreak.html.

6. Shamane Mills, "Delta 'Opened the Door': Rural Deaths from COVID-19 Now Higher than in Urban Areas," *Wisconsin Public Radio*, October 13, 2021,

https://www.wpr.org/delta-opened-door-rural-deaths-covid-19-now-higher-urban-areas.

7. Farah Stockman et al., "'They're Death Pits': Virus Claims at Least 7,000 Lives in U.S. Nursing Homes," *New York Times*, April 17, 2020, https://www.nytimes.com/2020/04/17/us/coronavirus-nursing-homes.html.

8. Danny Hakim, "'It's Hit Our Front Door': Homes for the Disabled See a Surge of Covid-19," *New York Times*, April 8, 2020, https://www.nytimes.com/2020/04/08/nyregion/coronavirus-disabilities-group-homes.html.

9. Women in healthcare have found more opportunities in recent decades in well-paying jobs like surgeons and physicians, but women, "have also been filling the unseen jobs proliferating on the lowest end of the wage scale, the workers who spend long and little-rewarded days bathing, feeding and medicating some of the most vulnerable people in the country. Of the 5.8 million people working health care jobs that pay less than $30,000 a year, half are nonwhite and 83 percent are women." See Campbell Robertson and Robert Gebeloff, "How Millions of Women Became the Most Essential Workers in America," *New York Times*, April 18, 2020, https://www.nytimes.com/2020/04/18/us/coronavirus-women-essential-workers.html.

10. Richard Lee, *The Dobe Ju/'Hoansi*, 4th ed. (Belmont, CA: Wadsworth Cengage Learning, 2012), 104.

11. Laurel White and Rich Kremer, "Wisconsin Supreme Court Strikes Down Statewide Mask Mandate," *Wisconsin Public Radio*, March 30, 2021, https://www.wpr.org/wisconsin-supreme-court-strikes-down-statewide-mask-mandate.

12. County officials also recommended other layers of mitigation, including vaccination of those eligible, physical distancing, use of quarantine measures, testing, ventilation, and handwashing.

13. Ashley Kieran Clift et al., "COVID-19 Mortality Risk in Down Syndrome: Results From a Cohort Study of 8 Million Adults," *Annals of Internal Medicine* 174, no. 4 (April 20, 2021): 572–76, https://doi.org/10.7326/M20-4986; David Emes et al., "COVID-19 in Children with Down Syndrome: Data from the Trisomy 21 Research Society Survey," *MedRxiv*, July 2, 2021, https://doi.org/10.1101/2021.06.25.21259525; Julia Hippisley-Cox et al., "Risk Prediction of Covid-19 Related Death and Hospital Admission in Adults after Covid-19 Vaccination: National Prospective Cohort Study," *BMJ* 374 (September 17, 2021): n2244, https://doi.org/10.1136/bmj.n2244; Anke Hüls et al., "Medical Vulnerability of Individuals with Down Syndrome to Severe COVID-19—Data from the Trisomy 21 Research Society and the UK ISARIC4C Survey," *EClinicalMedicine* 33 (March 1, 2021), https://doi.org/10.1016/j.eclinm.2021.100769; Meredith Wadman, "People with Down Syndrome Face High Risk from Coronavirus," *Science* 370, no. 6523 (December 18, 2020): 1384–85.

14. Wadman, "People with Down Syndrome Face High Risk from Coronavirus."

15. In a context where other mitigation measures are used, such as frequent testing and widespread vaccination, masks could be unnecessary, or at least a safety measure of last resort. But the Delta variant altered the calculus, with increasing rates of infection among children as the school year commenced around the country. Plus, widespread vaccine hesitancy had left rural communities especially vulnerable, and the vaccine was not yet approved for children under twelve years old. Given such conditions, universal masking seemed an easy and low-cost mitigation strategy to try to keep kids safe and in school, at least until vaccines were available to all age groups. This was the reasoning of public health officials and the school district leadership. For an argument opposed to masking as a mitigation measure in schools, see Marty Makary and H. Cody Meissner, "The Case against Masks for Children," *Wall Street Journal*, August 8, 2021, https://www.wsj.com/articles/masks-children-parenting-schools-mandates-covid-19-coronavirus-pandemic-biden-administration-cdc-11628432716.

16. Sean B. Carroll, "The Denialist Playbook," *Scientific American*, November 8, 2020, https://www.scientificamerican.com/article/the-denialist-playbook/.

17. Under Section 504 of the Rehabilitation Act of 1973 and Title II of the Americans with Disabilities Act (ADA), schools must provide reasonable accommodations to ensure equal access to public education.

18. Doron Raz and Doron Dorfman, "Students with Disabilities Could Sue Their Schools to Require Masks," *Washington Post*, August 19, 2021, https://www.washingtonpost.com/outlook/2021/08/19/school-masking-americans-disability-act/; Mical Raz and Doron Dorfman, "Bans on COVID-19 Mask Requirements vs Disability Accommodations: A New Conundrum," *JAMA Health Forum* 2, no. 8 (August 6, 2021): e211912, https://doi.org/10.1001/jamahealthforum.2021.1912.

19. U.S. Department of Education Press Office, "Department of Education's Office for Civil Rights Opens Investigations in Five States Regarding Prohibitions of Universal Indoor Masking," news release, August 30, 2021, https://www.ed.gov/news/press-releases/department-educations-office-civil-rights-opens-investigations-five-states-regarding-prohibitions-universal-indoor-masking.

20. Lewis A. Grossman, "The Origins of American Health Libertarianism," *Yale Journal of Health Policy, Law, and Ethics* 13, no. 1 (2013): 80.

21. Grossman, "Origins of American Health Libertarianism," 80.

22. "Alternative medicine movements continued to arise throughout the twentieth century," writes Grossman, producing "a kaleidoscope of theories and philosophies" that clustered around similar attitudes such as "skepticism toward orthodox medical science, an embrace of more 'natural' and lower-risk

alternatives to regular drugs, and, in many instances, a populist suspicion of nefarious conspiracies involving the medical elite." See Grossman, 128.

23. Peter J. Hotez, "America's Deadly Flirtation with Antiscience and the Medical Freedom Movement," *Journal of Clinical Investigation* 131, no. 7 (April 1, 2021): 2, https://doi.org/10.1172/JCI149072.

24. Maggie Astor, "Vaccination Mandates Are an American Tradition. So Is the Backlash," *New York Times*, September 9, 2021, https://www.nytimes.com/2021/09/09/us/politics/vaccine-mandates-history.html.

25. Hotez, "America's Deadly Flirtation," 1.

26. Lewis A. Grossman, *Choose Your Medicine: Freedom of Therapeutic Choice in America* (Oxford: Oxford University Press, 2021).

27. Hotez, "America's Deadly Flirtation," 2.

28. Roy Richard Grinker, *Unstrange Minds: Remapping the World of Autism* (New York: Basic Books, 2007).

29. Hotez, "America's Deadly Flirtation," 2.

30. Hotez, 2.

31. Susannah Crockford, "The 'Health Freedom Movement' Enters the Covid Era by Disseminating Medical Disinformation," *Religion Dispatches*, May 13, 2021, https://religiondispatches.org/the-health-freedom-movement-enters-the-covid-era-by-disseminating-medical-disinformation/.

32. Crockford, "Health Freedom Movement'."

33. Crockford.

34. Emily Martin, *Flexible Bodies: Tracking Immunity in American Culture: From the Days of Polio to the Age of AIDS* (Boston: Beacon Press, 1994).

35. Maggie Astor, "Vocal Anti-Vaccine Chiropractors Split the Profession," *New York Times*, July 14, 2021, https://www.nytimes.com/2021/07/14/health/anti-covid-vaxxers.html.

36. Michelle R. Smith, Scott Bauer, and Mike Catalini, "Anti-Vaccine Chiropractors Rising Force of Misinformation," *AP*, October 8, 2021, https://apnews.com/article/anti-virus-chiropractors-rising-force-misinformation-02b347767b45cab1d6d532be03c57529.

37. Chiropractic Society of Wisconsin, "Health Freedom Revival—Billy DeMoss," Facebook, video, August 19, 2021, https://www.facebook.com/chiropracticsocietywi/videos/health-freedom-revival-billy-demoss/202674128504582/.

38. Center for Countering Digital Hate, "The Disinformation Dozen," March 21, 2021, https://www.counterhate.com/disinformationdozen.

39. In addition to such experts, the Health Freedom Revivals featured self-described "warrior moms" protesting mask requirements and vaccine mandates, who shared stories in which they overcame the threat of mainstream medicine to achieve personal growth and wellbeing. The one actual medical doctor in the speaker lineup was pediatrician Robert Zajac of New Kingdom Healthcare,

billed as "an expert in vaccine safety and holistic care." Zajac had recently been disciplined by the Minnesota Board of Medical Practice for telling parents that childhood vaccines are unsafe. See Glenn Howatt, "Minnesota Pediatrician Disciplined for Discouraging Childhood Vaccines," *Star Tribune*, August 11, 2021, https://www.startribune.com/minnesota-pediatrician-disciplined-for-discouraging-childhood-vaccines/600087021/.

40. Crockford, "Health Freedom Movement."

41. Moses's testimony on AB309 was given at a public hearing of the Assembly Committee on Constitution and Ethics, in Madison, on June 2, 2021. A video of the testimony is available on his campaign Facebook page: Representative Clint Moses, "Yesterday I gave testimony on my bill AB309 which prohibits discrimination based on vaccination status. There were many people. . .," Facebook video, June 3, 2021, https://www.facebook.com/watch/?v=478552543410734.

42. Elizabeth Beyer and Lucas Robinson, "Fort Atkinson School Board Mandates Masks Following Death of 13-Year-Old Student," *Wisconsin State Journal*, September 18, 2021, https://madison.com/news/local/education/local_schools/fort-atkinson-school-board-mandates-masks-following-death-of-13-year-old-student/article_efc7e8e6-ccf6-5320-9e17-30aa3ed9fb94.html.

43. Julian Emerson, "A Mondovi High Schooler Died While COVID-Positive. The School Board Still Didn't Require Masks," *UpNorthNews*, September 24, 2021, https://upnorthnewswi.com/2021/09/24/a-mondovi-high-schooler-died-while-covid-positive-the-school-board-still-didnt-require-masks/.

44. Julian Emerson, "Parents, Progressive PAC Weigh Lawsuits against Schools That Refuse to Enact COVID Rules," *UpNorthNews*, September 27, 2021,https://upnorthnewswi.com/2021/09/27/parents-pac-weigh-lawsuits-against-schools-refuse-covid-rules/.

45. Eduardo Medina, "A Judge Says Texas' Ban on Mask Mandates Violates the Rights of Students with Disabilities.," *New York Times*, November 11, 2021, https://www.nytimes.com/2021/11/10/us/judge-rules-mandates-up-to-texas-schools.html.

46. Julian Emerson, "Menomonie Parents Request Due Process Hearing over School District's COVID Safety Protocols," *UpNorthNews*, October 2, 2021,https://upnorthnewswi.com/2021/10/02/menomonie-parents-request-due-process-hearing-over-school-districts-covid-safety-protocols/; Erik Gunn, "Parents Say Public Health Backlash Risks Their Child's Life," *Wisconsin Examiner*, October 2, 2021, https://wisconsinexaminer.com/2021/10/02/parents-the-public-health-backlash-risks-our-childs-life/.

47. Tom Shakespeare, *Disability: The Basics* (New York: Routledge, 2018), 50.

48. Tom Shakespeare, "Nasty, Brutish, and Short? On the Predicament of Disability and Embodiment," in *Disability and the Good Human Life*, ed. Jerome E. Bickenbach, Franziska Felder, and Barbara Schmitz (New York: Cambridge University Press, 2014), 109.

49. Eva Feder Kittay, "Centering Justice on Dependency and Recovering Freedom," *Hypatia* 30, no. 1 (2015): 285–91, https://doi.org/10.1111/hypa.12131; Eva Feder Kittay, *Learning from My Daughter: The Value and Care of Disabled Minds* (Oxford: Oxford University Press, 2019).

EPILOGUE

1. Rosemarie Garland-Thomson, "The Case for Conserving Disability," *Bioethical Inquiry* 9, no. 3 (2012): 342.

2. Garland-Thomson writes of six truths: "All human beings need care, assistance, and a sustaining environment to life; disability disadvantage results from living in an unaccommodating environment; quality of life cannot be predicted in advance; disability can produce life advantages; what counts as disability changes over time and space; and the border between disabled and nondisabled shifts over a lifetime." See Rosemarie Garland-Thomson, "Human Biodiversity Conservation: A Consensual Ethical Principle," *American Journal of Bioethics* 15, no. 6 (June 2015): 15, https://doi.org/10.1080/15265161.2015.1028663.

3. Erin L. Durban, "Anthropology and Ableism," *American Anthropologist* 124, no. 1 (2022): 8–20, https://doi.org/10.1111/aman.13659.

4. Danilyn Rutherford, "Proximity to Disability," *Anthropological Quarterly* 93, no. 1 (2020): 1453–81.

5. Tom Shakespeare, *Disability: The Basics* (New York: Routledge, 2018), 22.

6. For a powerful illustration of this, see Sunaura Taylor, *Beasts of Burden: Animal and Disability Liberation* (New York: New Press, 2017).

Bibliography

Adams, Rachel. *Raising Henry: A Memoir of Motherhood, Disability, and Discovery.* New Haven, CT: Yale University Press, 2013.

Allen, Gordon, C. E. Benda, J. A. Böök, C. O. Carter, C. E. Ford, E. H. Y. Chu, E. Hanhart, et al. "Mongolism." *American Journal of Human Genetics* 13, no. 4 (1961): 426.

———. "Mongolism." *The Lancet* 277, no. 7180 (1961): 775.

Annas, George J. "Denying the Rights of the Retarded: The Phillip Becker Case." *Hastings Center Report* 9, no. 6 (1979): 18–20. https://doi.org/10.2307/3561672.

Austin, Paul. *Beautiful Eyes: A Father Transformed.* New York: W. W. Norton, 2014.

Ayrault, Evelyn West. *You Can Raise Your Handicapped Child.* New York: G. P. Putnam's Sons, 1964.

Baker, Lee D. *From Savage to Negro: Anthropology and the Construction of Race, 1896–1954.* Berkeley: University of California Press, 1998.

———. "The Racist Anti-Racism of American Anthropology." *Transforming Anthropology* 290, no. 2 (2020): 127–42.

Benedict, Ruth. "Anthropology and the Abnormal." *Journal of General Psychology* 10, no. 1 (1934): 59–82.

Berliner, Alan, dir. *Margaret Mead: An Observer Observed.* New York: Filmakers Library, 1996.

Bérubé, Michael. "Equality, Freedom, and/or Justice for All: A Response to Martha Nussbaum." *Metaphilosophy* 40, no. 3/4 (2009): 352–65.

———. *Life as Jamie Knows It: An Exceptional Child Grows Up.* Boston: Beacon Press, 2016.

———. *Life as We Know It: A Father, a Family, and an Exceptional Child.* New York: Vintage Books, 1998.

Blatt, Burton, and Fred Kaplan. *Christmas in Purgatory: A Photographic Essay on Mental Retardation.* Syracuse, NY: Human Policy Press, 1974.

Bloland, Sue Erikson. *In the Shadow of Fame: A Memoir by the Daughter of Erik H. Erikson.* New York: Viking, 2006.

Campbell, Fiona Kumari. *Contours of Ableism: The Production of Disability and Abledness.* New York: Palgrave Macmillan, 2009.

Carey, Allison C. *On the Margins of Citizenship: Intellectual Disability and Civil Rights in Twentieth-Century America.* Philadelphia: Temple University Press, 2010.

Carey, Allison C., Pamela Block, and Richard Scotch. *Allies and Obstacles: Disability Activism and Parents of Children with Disabilities.* Philadelphia: Temple University Press, 2020.

Clift, Ashley Kieran, Carol A. C. Coupland, Ruth H. Keogh, Harry Hemingway, and Julia Hippisley-Cox. "COVID-19 Mortality Risk in Down Syndrome: Results from a Cohort Study of 8 Million Adults." *Annals of Internal Medicine* 174, no. 4 (2021): 572–76. https://doi.org/10.7326/M20-4986.

Cohen, Adam Seth. *Imbeciles: The Supreme Court, American Eugenics, and the Sterilization of Carrie Buck.* New York: Penguin Press, 2016.

Cohen, Deborah. 2013. *Family Secrets: Shame and Privacy in Modern Britain.* Oxford: Oxford University Press, 2013.

Cooney, Joan Ganz. "Foreword." In *Count Us In: Growing Up with Down Syndrome,* viii–x. Orlando, FL: Mariner Books, 2007.

Crookshank, Francis Graham. *The Mongol in Our Midst: A Study of Man and His Three Faces.* New York: E. P. Dutton, 1924.

Davis, Lennard J. *Enabling Acts: The Hidden Story of How the Americans with Disability Act Gave the Largest U.S. Minority Its Rights.* Boston: Beacon Press, 2016.

———. "Introduction: Disability, Normality, and Power." In *The Disability Studies Reader,* edited by Lennard J. Davis, 5th ed., 1–14. New York: Routledge, 2017.

Dolmage, Jay T. *Academic Ableism: Disability and Higher Education.* Ann Arbor: University of Michigan Press, 2017.

Dougan, Terrell Harris. *That Went Well: Adventures in Caring for My Sister.* New York: Hachette Books, 2009.

Down, John Langdon H. "Observations on an Ethnic Classification of Idiots." *London Hospital Reports* 3 (1866): 259–62.

Durban, Erin L. "Anthropology and Ableism." *American Anthropologist* 124, no. 1 (2022): 8–20. https://doi.org/10.1111/aman.13659.

Emes, David, Anke Hüls, Nicole Baumer, Mara Dierssen, Shiela Puri, Lauren Russel, Stephanie L. Sherman, et al. "COVID-19 in Children with Down Syndrome: Data from the Trisomy 21 Research Society Survey." *MedRxiv*, July 2, 2021. https://doi.org/10.1101/2021.06.25.21259525.

Erevelles, Nirmala, and Andrea Minear. "Unspeakable Offenses: Untangling Race and Disability in Discourses of Intersectionality." *Journal of Literacy and Cultural Disability Studies* 4, no. 2 (2010): 127–45.

Estreich, George. *Fables and Futures: Biotechnology, Disability, and the Stories We Tell Ourselves.* Cambridge, MA: MIT Press, 2019.

———. *The Shape of the Eye: A Memoir.* New York: Penguin, 2013.

Farmer, Paul. "An Anthropology of Structural Violence." *Current Anthropology* 45, no. 3 (2004): 305–25. https://doi.org/10.1086/382250.

———. "On Suffering and Structural Violence: A View from Below." *Daedalus* 125, no. 1 (1996): 261–83.

Farmer, Paul E., Bruce Nizeye, Sara Stulac, and Salmaan Keshavjee. "Structural Violence and Clinical Medicine." *PLOS Medicine* 3, no. 10 (2006): 1686–91. https://doi.org/10.1371/journal.pmed.0030449.

Fost, Norman. "'The Hopkins Mongol Case': The Dawn of the Bioethics Movement." *Pediatrics* 146, no. s1 (2020): s3–8.

Freeman, Victoria. *A World without Martha: A Memoir of Sisters, Disability, and Difference.* Vancouver: University of British Columbia Press, 2019.

Friedman, Lawrence Jacob. *Identity's Architect: A Biography of Erik H. Erikson.* Cambridge, MA: Harvard University Press, 2000.

Galton, Francis. *Inquiries into Human Faculty and Its Development.* London: Macmillan, 1883.

Garland-Thomson, Rosemarie. "The Case for Conserving Disability." *Bioethical Inquiry* 9, no. 3 (2012): 339–55.

———. "A Habitable World: Harriet McBryde Johnson's 'Case for My Life.'" *Hypatia* 30, no. 1 (2015): 300–306.

———. "Human Biodiversity Conservation: A Consensual Ethical Principle." *American Journal of Bioethics* 15, no. 6 (2015): 13–15. https://doi.org/10.10 80/15265161.2015.1028663.

———. *Staring: How We Look.* New York: Oxford University Press, 2009.

Gelb, Steven A. "Darwin's Use of Intellectual Disability in *The Descent of Man*." *Disability Studies Quarterly* 28, no. 2 (2008). https://doi.org/10.18061/dsq .v28i2.96.

Ginsburg, Faye D., and Rayna Rapp. "Cognitive Disability: Towards an Ethics of Possibility." *Cambridge Journal of Anthropology* 36, no. 1 (2018): 113–19.

———, eds. *Conceiving the New World Order: The Global Politics of Reproduction.* Berkeley: University of California Press, 1995.

——. "Disability/Anthropology: Rethinking the Parameters of the Human: An Introduction to Supplement 21." *Current Anthropology* 61, no. s21 (2020): s4–15.

——. "Disability Worlds." *Annual Review of Anthropology* 42 (2013): 53–68.

——. "Entangled Ethnography: Imagining a Future for Young Adults with Learning Disabilities." *Social Science and Medicine* 99 (December 2013): 187–93. https://doi.org/10.1016/j.socscimed.2013.11.015.

Goc, Michael J., ed. *Island of Refuge: The Northern Wisconsin Center for the Developmentally Disabled, 1897–1997*. Friendship, WI: New Past Press, 1997.

Goddard, Henry Herbert. *The Kallikak Family: A Study in the Heredity of Feeblemindedness*. New York: Macmillan, 1921.

Goffman, Erving. "Interpersonal Persuasion." In *Group Processes: Transactions of the Third Conference*, edited by Bertram Schaffner, 117–93. New York: Madison Printing Company, 1957.

Gould, Stephen Jay. *The Mismeasure of Man*. New York: W. W. Norton, 1996.

Grant, Madison. *The Passing of the Great Race: Or, The Racial Basis of European History*. New York: Charles Scribner's Sons, 1918.

Grinker, Roy Richard. *Nobody's Normal: How Culture Created the Stigma of Mental Illness*. New York: W. W. Norton, 2021.

——. *Unstrange Minds: Remapping the World of Autism*. New York: Basic Books, 2007.

Grossman, Lewis A. *Choose Your Medicine: Freedom of Therapeutic Choice in America*. Oxford: Oxford University Press, 2021.

——. "The Origins of American Health Libertarianism." *Yale Journal of Health Policy, Law, and Ethics* 13, no. 1 (2013): 76–134.

Gwaltney, John Langston. "The Blind of San Pedro Yolox." *The American Scholar* 35, no. 1 (1965): 114–25.

——. "Some Thoughts on Native Anthropology." *Transforming Anthropology* 7, no. 2 (1998): 67–69.

——. *The Thrice Shy: Cultural Accommodation to Blindness and Other Disasters in a Mexican Community*. New York: Columbia University Press, 1970.

Hippisley-Cox, Julia, Carol A. C. Coupland, Nisha Mehta, Ruth H. Keogh, Karla Diaz-Ordaz, Kamlesh Khunti, Ronan A. Lyons, et al. "Risk Prediction of Covid-19 Related Death and Hospital Admission in Adults after Covid-19 Vaccination: National Prospective Cohort Study." *BMJ* 374 (September 2021): n2244. https://doi.org/10.1136/bmj.n2244.

Hotez, Peter J. "America's Deadly Flirtation with Antiscience and the Medical Freedom Movement." *Journal of Clinical Investigation* 131, no. 7 (2021): 1–3. https://doi.org/10.1172/JCI149072.

Hüls, Anke, Alberto C. S. Costa, Mara Dierssen, R. Asaad Baksh, Stefania Bargagna, Nicole T. Baumer, Ana Claudia Brandão, et al. "Medical Vulnerability of Individuals with Down Syndrome to Severe COVID-19—Data from the Trisomy 21 Research Society and the UK ISARIC4C Survey." *EClinicalMedicine* 33 (March 2021). https://doi.org/10.1016/j.eclinm.2021.100769.

Jackson, Aaron J. *Worlds of Care: The Emotional Lives of Fathers Caring for Children with Disabilities.* Oakland: University of California Press, 2021.

Kafer, Alison. *Feminist, Queer, Crip.* Bloomington: Indiana University Press, 2013.

Kaposy, Chris. *Choosing Down Syndrome: Ethics and New Prenatal Testing Technologies.* Cambridge, MA: MIT Press, 2018.

Keevak, Michael. *Becoming Yellow: A Short History of Racial Thinking.* Princeton, NJ: Princeton University Press, 2011.

King, Charles. *Gods of the Upper Air: How a Circle of Renegade Anthropologists Reinvented Race, Sex, and Gender in the Twentieth Century.* New York: Anchor Books, 2019.

Kittay, Eva Feder. "Centering Justice on Dependency and Recovering Freedom." *Hypatia* 30, no. 1 (2015): 285–91. https://doi.org/10.1111/hypa.12131.

———. "Forever Small: The Strange Case of Ashley X." *Hypatia* 26, no. 3 (2011): 610–31. https://doi.org/10.1111/j.1527-2001.2011.01205.x.

———. *Learning from My Daughter: The Value and Care of Disabled Minds.* Oxford?: Oxford University Press, 2019.

Kuhse, Helga, and Peter Singer. *Should the Baby Live? The Problem of Handicapped Infants.* New York: Oxford University Press, 1985.

La Barre, Weston. "Review of 'Psychological and Cultural Problems in Mental Subnormality: A Review of Research,' by Seymour B. Sarason and Thomas Gladwin." *American Anthropologist* 61, no. 1 (1959): 166–67.

Landsman, Gail. *Reconstructing Motherhood and Disability in the Age of Perfect Babies.* New York: Routledge, 2008.

Lee, Richard. *The Dobe Ju/'Hoansi.* 4th ed. Belmont, CA: Wadsworth Cengage Learning, 2012.

Leonard, Thomas C. *Illiberal Reformers: Race, Eugenics, and American Economics in the Progressive Era.* Princeton, NJ: Princeton University Press, 2016.

Mandler, Peter. *Return from the Natives: How Margaret Mead Won the Second World War and Lost the Cold War.* New Haven, CT: Yale University Press, 2013.

Martin, Emily. *Flexible Bodies: Tracking Immunity in American Culture: From the Days of Polio to the Age of AIDS.* Boston: Beacon Press, 1994.

Masland, Richard L., Seymour B. Sarason, and Thomas Gladwin. *Mental Subnormality: Biological, Psychological, and Cultural Factors.* New York: Basic Books, 1958.

McKearney, Patrick, and Tyler Zoanni. "Introduction: For an Anthropology of Cognitive Disability." *Cambridge Journal of Anthropology* 36, no. 1 (2018): 1–22.

Mead, Margaret. *Coming of Age in Samoa*. Laurel ed. New York: Dell Publishing Company, 1968 [1928].

———. *Culture and Commitment: A Study of the Generation Gap*. New York: Doubleday, 1970.

———. "Dr. Margaret Mead's Address." In *Annual Meeting Minutes: The President's Committee on Employment of the Handicapped*, 7–9. Washington, DC: Bureau of Labor Standards, 1967.

———. "Research: Cult or Cure?" *American Journal of Mental Deficiency* 64 (1959): 253–64.

———. "Statement of Dr. Margaret Mead to the 1969 Joint Commission on Mental Health of Children." In *Departments of Labor, Health and Human Services, Education, and Related Agencies Appropriations for 1984; Hearings Before a Subcommittee of the Committee on Appropriations, House of Representatives, Ninety-Eighth Congress, First Session; Part 8, Testimony of Members of Congress and Interested Individuals and Organizations*. Washington, DC: U.S. Government Printing Office, 1983.

Newton, Esther. *Margaret Mead Made Me Gay: Personal Essays, Public Ideas*. Durham, NC: Duke University Press, 2000.

Nielsen, Kim E. *A Disability History of the United States*. Boston: Beacon Press, 2012.

Noonan, Jacqueline A. "A History of Pediatric Specialties: The Development of Pediatric Cardiology." *Pediatric Research* 56, no. 2 (2004): 298–306. https://doi.org/10.1203/01.PDR.0000132662.73362.96.

Ochs, Elinor, and Olga Solomon. "Autistic Sociality." *Ethos* 38, no. 1 (2010): 69–92.

Opler, Marvin K. "Review of 'Mental Subnormality: Biological, Psychological and Cultural Factors,' by Richard L. Masland, Seymour B. Sarason, and Thomas Gladwin." *American Anthropologist* 61, no. 6 (1959): 1160–61.

Parens, Erik, and Adrienne Asch. "The Disability Rights Critique of Prenatal Genetic Testing: Reflections and Recommendations." *Hastings Center Report* 29, no. 5 (1999): s1–22.

Piepmeier, Alison. *Unexpected: Parenting, Prenatal Testing, and Down Syndrome*. With George Estreich and Rachel Adams. New York: NYU Press, 2021.

Rapp, Emily. *The Still Point of the Turning World*. New York: Penguin, 2014.

Rapp, Rayna. "After Mead." In "Margaret Mead's Legacy: Continuing Conversations." Special issue, *Scholar and Feminist Online* 1, no. 2 (2003). http://sfonline.barnard.edu/mead/rapp.htm.

———. *Testing Women, Testing the Fetus: The Social Impact of Amniocentesis in America*. New York: Routledge, 2000.

Rapp, Rayna, and Faye Ginsburg. "Reverberations: Disability and the New Kinship Imaginary." *Anthropological Quarterly* 84, no. 2 (2011): 379–410.

Raz, Mical, and Doron Dorfman. "Bans on COVID-19 Mask Requirements vs Disability Accommodations: A New Conundrum." *JAMA Health Forum* 2, no. 8 (2021): e211912. https://doi.org/10.1001/jamahealthforum.2021 .1912.

Reno, Joshua, Kaitlyn Hart, Amy Mendelson, and Felicia Molzon. "Toward a Critical and Comparative Anthropology of Disability: Absent Presence and Exemplary Personhood." *Social Analysis* 65, no. 3 (2021): 131–49. https:// doi.org/10.3167/sa.2021.650307.

Rutherford, Danilyn. "Proximity to Disability." *Anthropological Quarterly* 93, no. 1 (2020): 1453–81.

Sandel, Michael J. *The Case against Perfection: Ethics in the Age of Genetic Engineering.* Cambridge, MA: Belknap Press, 2007.

Sarason, Seymour B., and Thomas Gladwin. "Psychological and Cultural Problems in Mental Subnormality." *Genetic Psychology Monographs* 57 (1958): 3–289.

Shakespeare, Tom. *Disability: The Basics.* New York: Routledge, 2018.

———. "Nasty, Brutish, and Short? On the Predicament of Disability and Embodiment." In *Disability and the Good Human Life,* edited by Jerome E. Bickenbach, Franziska Felder, and Barbara Schmitz, 93–112. New York: Cambridge University Press, 2014.

Shankman, Paul. "The Public Anthropology of Margaret Mead: *Redbook,* Women's Issues, and the 1960s." *Current Anthropology* 59, no. 1 (2018): 55–73.

Sharp, Lesley A. "The Ethnographic Vision of John L. Gwaltney: *The Thrice Shy,* A Forgotten Gem." *Somatosphere,* July 24, 2015. http://somatosphere .net/2015/the-ethnographic-vision-of-john-l-gwaltney-the-thrice-shy-a-forgotten-gem.html/.

Simpson, Audra. "Why White People Love Franz Boas; or, The Grammar of Indigenous Dispossession." In *Indigenous Visions: Rediscovering the World of Franz Boas,* edited by Ned Blackhawk and Isaiah Lorado Wilner, 166–81. New Haven, CT: Yale University Press, 2018.

Singer, Peter. *Rethinking Life and Death: The Collapse of Our Traditional Ethics.* New York: St. Martin's Griffin, 1994.

Solomon, Andrew. *Far from the Tree: Parents, Children, and the Search for Identity.* New York: Simon and Schuster, 2012.

Spiro, Jonathan Peter. *Defending the Master Race: Conservation, Eugenics, and the Legacy of Madison Grant.* Lebanon, NH: University Press of New England, 2009.

Stein, David S. *Supporting Positive Behavior in Children and Teens with Down Syndrome: The Respond but Don't React Method.* Bethesda, MD: Woodbine House, 2016.

"Subject Syllabi in Home and Social Economics, 1913–14: Eugenics." Stout Small Series 2, Vol. 3. 1913. The Stout Institute, University Archives and Area Research Center, University of Wisconsin-Stout.

Taylor, Sunaura. *Beasts of Burden: Animal and Disability Liberation.* New York: New Press, 2017.

Thomas, Gareth M. *Down's Syndrome Screening and Reproductive Politics: Care, Choice, and Disability in the Prenatal Clinic.* New York: Routledge, 2017.

———. "Un/Inhabitable Worlds: The Curious Case of Down's Syndrome." *Somatosphere,* July 29, 2015. http://somatosphere.net/2015/uninhabitable-worlds-the-curious-case-of-downs-syndrome.html/.

Tredgold, Alfred Frank, Roger Francis Tredgold, and Kenneth Soddy. *Textbook of Mental Deficiency (Subnormality).* Baltimore: Williams and Wilkins, 1963.

Trent, James W. *Inventing the Feeble Mind: A History of Mental Retardation in the United States.* Berkeley: University of California Press, 1994.

Volpe, E. Peter. "Is Down Syndrome a Modern Disease?" *Perspectives in Biology and Medicine* 29, no. 3-1 (1986): 423–36.

Wadman, Meredith. "People with Down Syndrome Face High Risk from Coronavirus." *Science* 370, no. 6523 (December 18, 2020): 1384–85. https://doi.org/10.1126/science.370.6523.1384.

Ward, O Conor. "John Langdon Down: The Man and the Message." *Down Syndrome Research and Practice* 6, no. 1 (1999): 19–24.

White, Michael. "The End at the Beginning." *Ochsner Journal* 11, no. 4 (2011): 309–16.

Wilmarth, A. W. "Heredity as a Social Burden." *Journal of the American Medical Association* 27, no. 7 (1896): 341–44.

———. "Superintendent's Report." In *Fifth Biennial Report of the Home for the Feeble-Minded, for the Biennial Period Ending June 30, 1906.* Madison: Democrat Printing, 1906.

———. "Superintendent's Report." In *Tenth Biennial Report of the Wisconsin Home for the Feeble-Minded, Located at Chippewa Falls, for the Biennial Period Ending June 30, 1916* Madison: State Board of Control of Wisconsin, 1916.

Wolfensberger, Wolf. "The Fiftieth Anniversary of What Appears to Be the World's First Doctoral Degree Program in Mental Retardation: Some Reminiscences of an Early Graduate." *Intellectual and Developmental Disabilities* 46, no. 1 (2008): 64–79.

———. *The Principle of Normalization in Human Services.* Toronto: National Institute on Mental Retardation, 1972.

Wright, David. *Downs: The History of a Disability.* New York: Oxford University Press, 2011.

———. "Mongols in Our Midst: John Langdon Down and the Ethnic Classification of Idiocy, 1858–1924." In *Mental Retardation in America: A Historical Reader,* edited by Steven Noll and James W. Trent, 92–119. New York: NYU Press, 2004.

Yanni, Carla. *The Architecture of Madness: Insane Asylums in the United States.* Minneapolis: University of Minnesota Press, 2007.

Index

Founded in 1893,
UNIVERSITY OF CALIFORNIA PRESS
publishes bold, progressive books and journals
on topics in the arts, humanities, social sciences,
and natural sciences—with a focus on social
justice issues—that inspire thought and action
among readers worldwide.

The UC PRESS FOUNDATION
raises funds to uphold the press's vital role
as an independent, nonprofit publisher, and
receives philanthropic support from a wide
range of individuals and institutions—and from
committed readers like you. To learn more, visit
ucpress.edu/supportus.